sattvic method
Awaken Conscious Wellbeing

Sattvic Sunrise

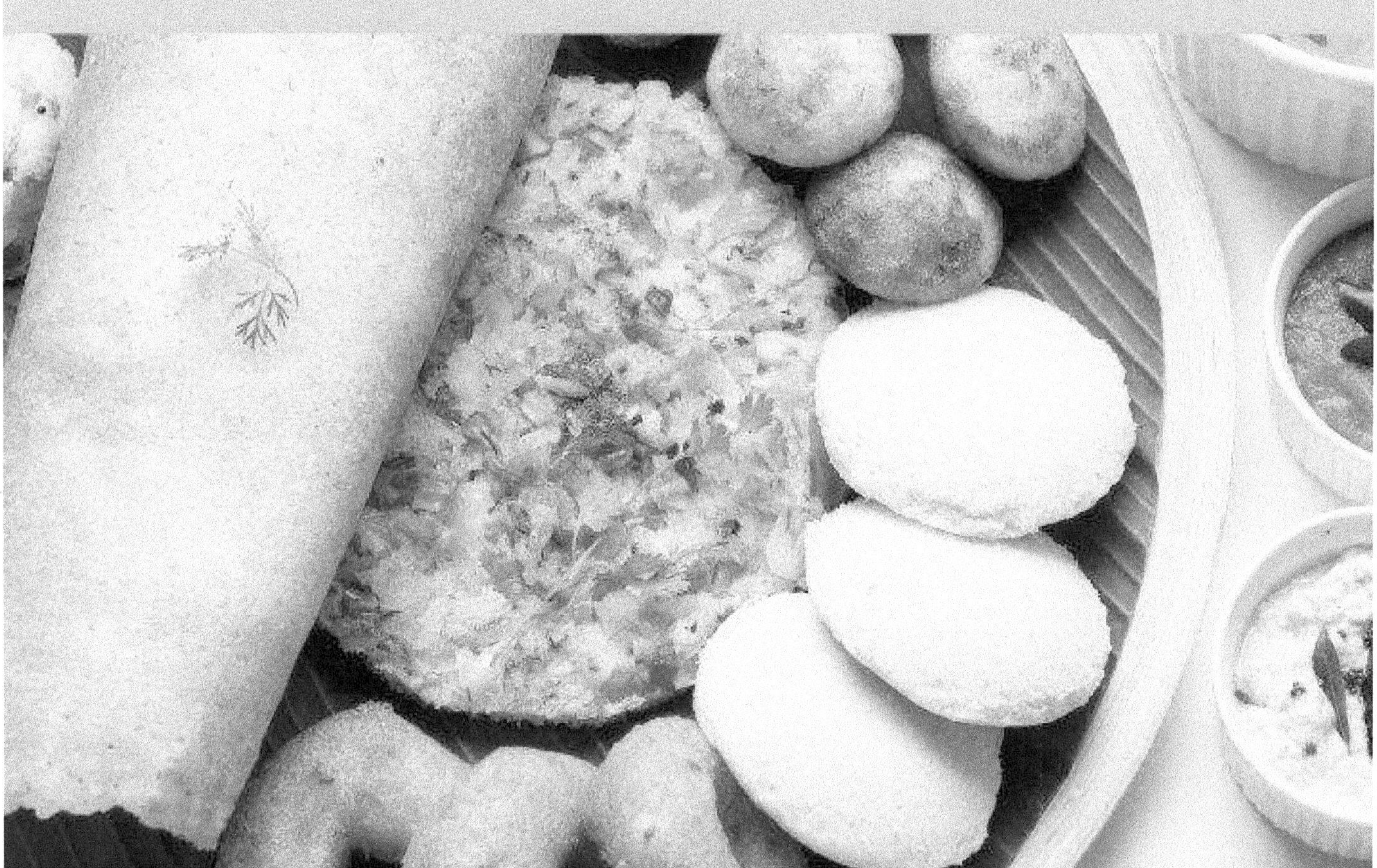

Wholesome South Indian Breakfasts for Holistic Wellness

© 2023 The Sattvic Method Company
All Rights Reserved

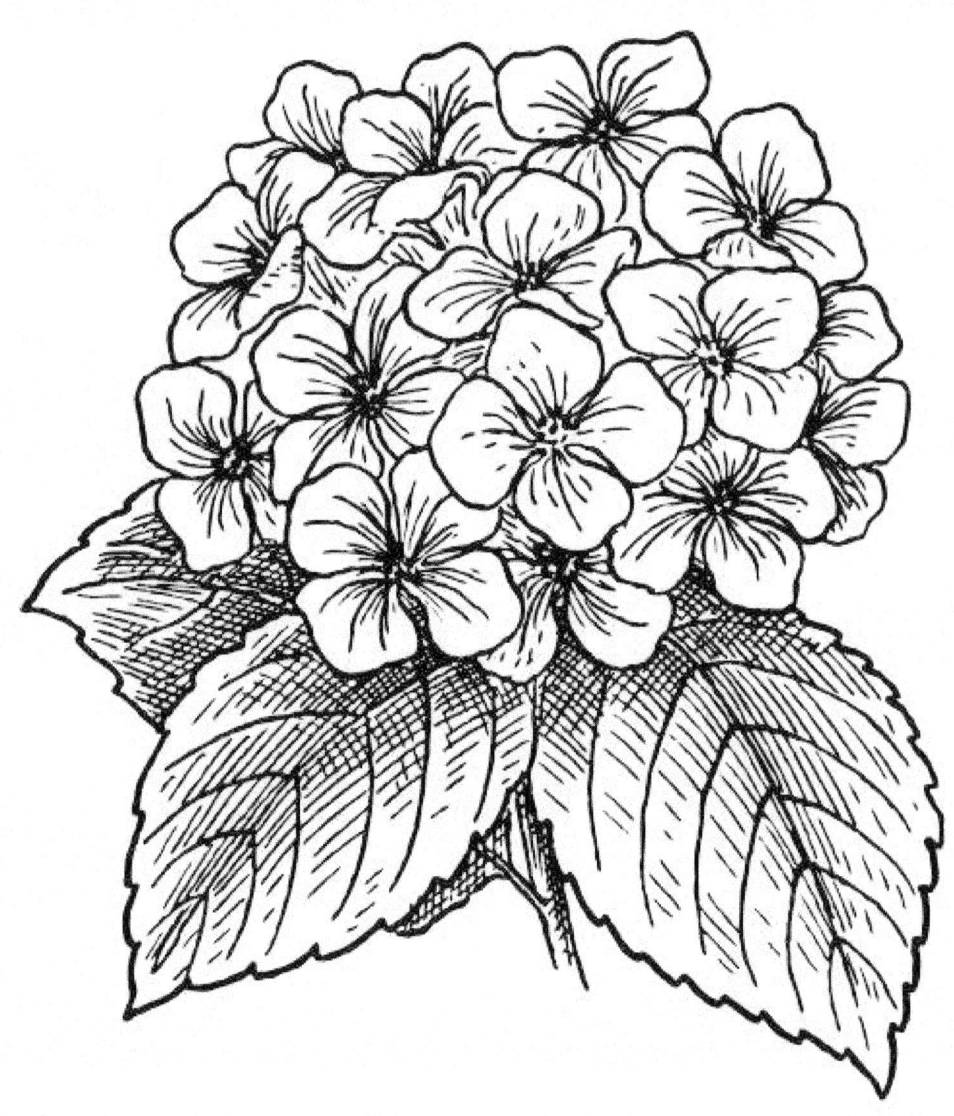

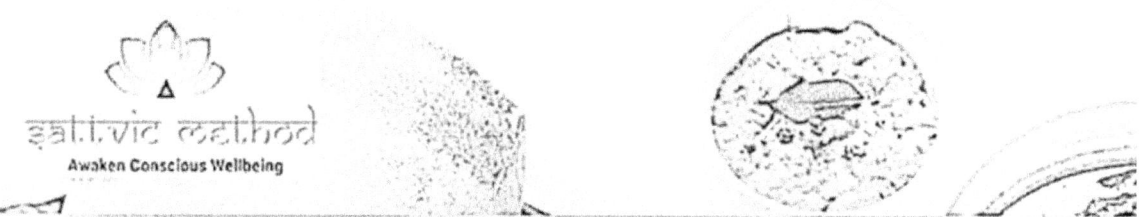

Sattvic Sunrise

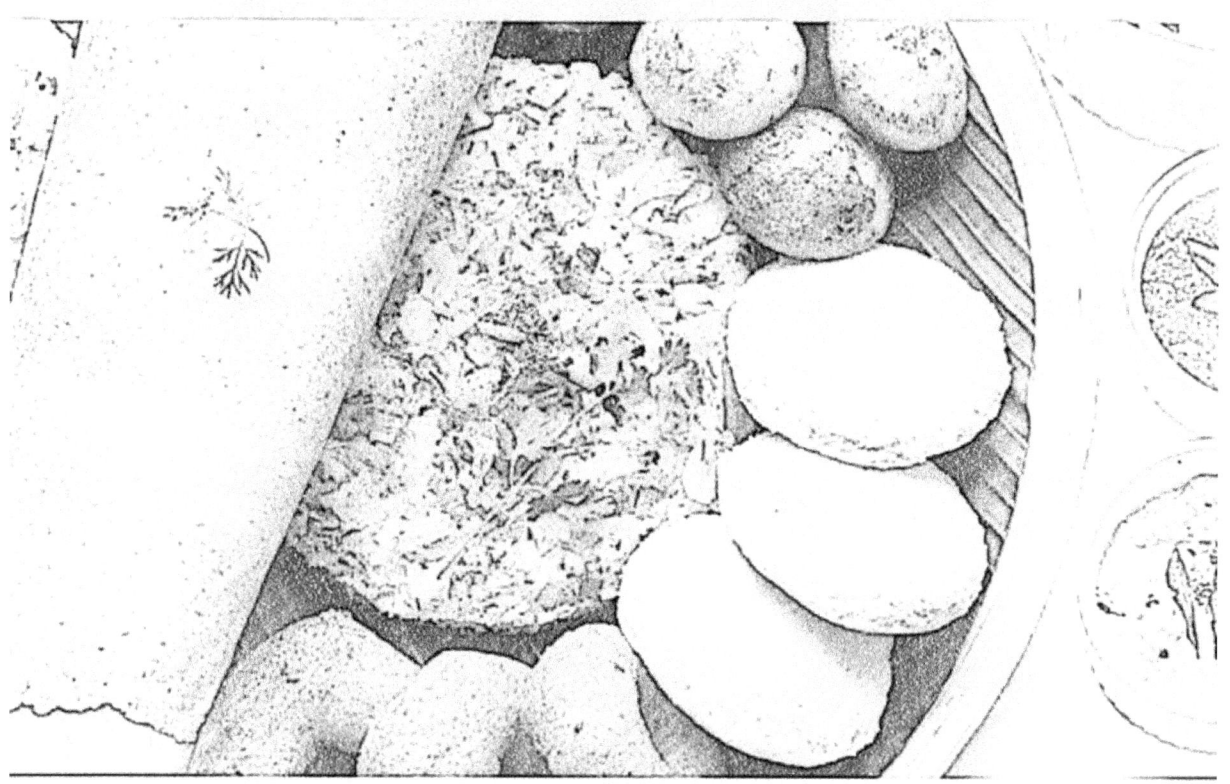

Wholesome South Indian Breakfasts for Holistic Wellness

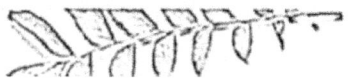

Discover the harmonious fusion of traditional South Indian flavors and Sattvic principles in 'Sattvic Sunrise,' your guide to nourishing morning meals that promote well-being and mindfulness.

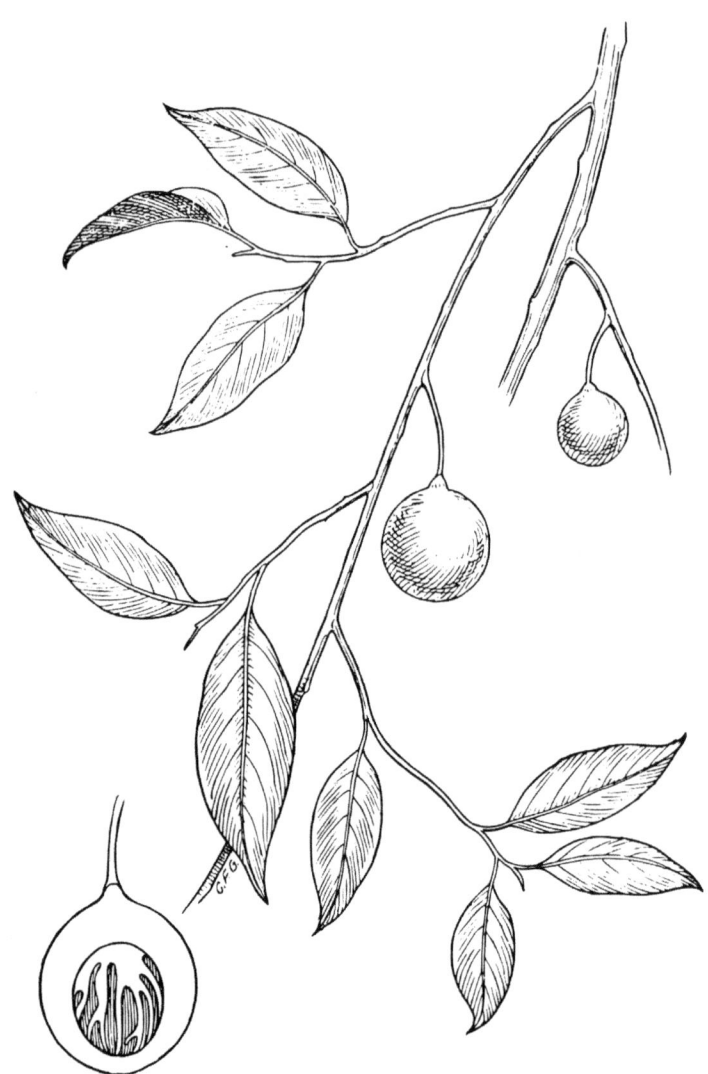

Contents

About Breakfast... 6
Sattvic Breakfast.. 9
About South Indian Cuisine.. 12
Importance of Preserving Traditional Breakfast... 15
   1. Adai.. 18
   2. Akki Roti.. 22
   3. Aapam.. 25
   4. Atho.. 29
   5. Aval Upma... 33
   6. Bisi Bele Baath.. 36
   7. Chana Sundal.. 40
   8. Coconut Rice... 44
   9. Dosa.. 47
   10. Idiyappam.. 50
   11. Karuveppilai Rice... 53
   12. Mangalore Buns.. 57
   13. Mango Rice... 60
   14. Masala Dosa.. 63
   15. Moong Dal Dosa... 67
   16. Neer Dosa.. 70
   17. Pazhampori.. 73
   18. Paniyaram.. 76
   19. Punugulu- Minapappu... 80
   20. Puttu... 83
   21. Rava Kesari... 86
   22. Rava idli.. 89
   21. Sevai... 92
   22. Thavalai Dosai.. 97
   23. Thayir Vadai... 101
   24. Tomato Upma... 106
   25. Uthappam.. 109
   26. Ven Pongal.. 113
   27. Vangibaath.. 116
   28. Wheat Rava Pongal... 120
   29. Yellu chadam.. 123
   30. Yelimichai Chadam... 127
List of ingredients used in the book... 130
Stocking your Sattvic Pantry... 132

About Breakfast

This book is about popular traditional South Indian breakfast recipes. It may include passing references about what our ancient Indian texts have to say. You may have picked up this book because you like eating South Indian food or because you are looking for alternate recipes to the oatmeal, bread, potatoes, eggs and bacon. You might be familiar with breakfast, lunch and dinner, plus snacks to keep you fueled up during the day, that is not the usual pattern of eating advised in the Sattvic Method.

Breakfast isn't directly mentioned in those old Vedic scriptures and shastras. However, they totally emphasize balanced meals and eating for wellbeing. The shastras however highlight the importance of timing your meals, choosing the right foods, and developing eating habits aligned with your requirement for the stage of life and to promote overall health. First, the Sattvic Method like Ayurveda is all about daily routines that help you to find balance. It supports you with precise and specific guidelines for when to eat, with regular mealtimes to aid digestion and keep your energy up. As you advance in the Sattvic Method, you can eat less and still perform efficiently.

The Sattvic Method has deep spiritual roots and recognizes the importance of the Brahma Muhurta that enables expansion of one's mind and being. It is the most precious time of the day, before dawn, and perfect for meditation, spiritual practices and setting yourself up for a positive day. Having a light, nourishing breakfast after meditating during Brahma Muhurta can provide energy and sustenance to fuel you for the rest of the day.

The shastras speak of Mitrahara moderation in eating. Consuming a balanced breakfast is key to avoid overeating later in the day. This aligns with the Sattvic Method and Ayurveda's advice to eat to satisfy hunger without overwhelming your digestive system. When you eat flavorful food mindfully you begin to experience a different level of fulfillment with the food, the mind, and the body.

Also, an important point to note is that- while breakfast isn't directly mentioned in the shastras, our ancient wisdom totally emphasizes balanced meals, including breakfast, for optimal wellbeing. The Shastras approach food with an energetic and conscious perspective as explained in detail in our upcoming book on Sattvic Weight Loss. What do you think? How can we embrace these teachings in our morning routines?

Here are some tips for successful Sattvic breakfast routines:

1. **Sattvic Diet:** The concept of a Sattvic diet, which includes foods that are considered pure, light, and harmonious, is rooted in shastras. Choosing Sattvic foods for breakfast can help maintain mental clarity, balance, and a sense of well-being. It can clear your brain fog or excessive reliance on coffee and other stimulants in the morning.
2. **Meal Timings:** While specific breakfast timings might not be mentioned, various texts discuss the importance of meal timings in relation to the body's natural rhythms and the digestive fire (agni). Eating breakfast within a reasonable time after waking up is seen as beneficial for jumpstarting metabolism and providing the body with necessary nutrients.
3. **Health and Longevity:** Many shastras emphasize the connection between diet and overall health. Consuming a balanced breakfast that includes a variety of nutrients can contribute to physical health, longevity, and vitality.

4. **Mind-Body Connection:** The shastras often recognize the interconnectedness of the mind and body. Having a nourishing breakfast can positively impact mental clarity, mood, and emotional well-being, aligning with the holistic approach of the shastras.

While the shastras provide guidance on various aspects of life, including diet and daily routines, it's important to interpret and apply their principles in a way that's relevant to modern times and individual needs. If you're interested in adopting specific dietary practices based on the shastras, you can sign up for guidance on our website thesattvicmethodcompany.com or choose to consult with experts in traditional Indian philosophy that can provide you with a more nuanced understanding and guidance.

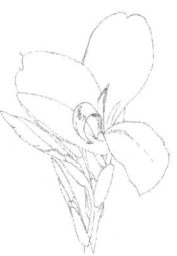

Sattvic Breakfast

Visualize this- you can begin your day with a light, life-positive supporting meal that keeps you feeling alert, active, and makes you feel hungry in about 3 or 4 hours. It does not take long to prepare and it gives you a reason to wake up 30 minutes early every day. After I moved to America, I struggled with bread and oatmeal for breakfast. The breakfast tasted insipid and worse, they left me bloated and with a stomach pain which sometimes seemed like hunger. Over the weekends when I made traditional breakfasts, I realized how much I missed the calming effect of drawing a dosa on the pan, and the aroma, texture, and the taste of food. Even the simple act of handling the food and breathing in the air when cooking the recipes gave me enormous satisfaction. This is the essence of Sattvic breakfast- a meal that aligns with the principles of Sattva, which is life-positive, engages and satisfies all your senses, and is so gentle on your system. Most of the South Indian breakfast recipes are made from fermented dough and when steamed or lightly cooked, they are very gentle on the stomach and gut.

The principles of the Sattvic Method come from the same roots of Ayurveda, an ancient Indian system of holistic health sciences, yoga, and mindfulness. Sattva is a quality of the food and is associated with purity, balance, and harmony, and eating energized sattvic breakfast is believed to promote natural intelligence and gentle qualities in both the body and mind. A Sattvic breakfast typically consists of foods that are light, easy to digest, and nourishing. Here are some potential advantages of consuming a Sattvic breakfast:

1. **Promotes Mental Clarity:** Sattvic foods are believed to have a calming and purifying effect on the mind. Consuming a Sattvic breakfast may help reduce mental agitation, promote clarity of thought, and improve focus.

2. **Balances Energy:** Sattvic foods are considered to be in harmony with nature and can provide a steady and balanced source of energy. They are not overly stimulating or heavy, which can help avoid energy crashes or feelings of lethargy after eating.

3. **Enhances Digestion:** Sattvic foods are typically easy to digest and gentle on the stomach. This can lead to improved digestion and less strain on the digestive system, allowing the body to absorb nutrients more effectively.

4. **Supports Emotional Well-being:** Ayurveda emphasizes the connection between food and emotions. Sattvic foods are thought to have a positive impact on emotions and mood, promoting a sense of calmness, happiness, and contentment.

5. **Maintains Physical Balance:** Sattvic foods are often plant-based and include fruits, vegetables, whole grains, nuts, and seeds. These foods provide essential nutrients, vitamins, and minerals, supporting overall physical health and well-being.

6. **Cleansing and Detoxifying:** Sattvic foods are often light and low in processed or artificial ingredients. This can contribute to a natural cleansing and detoxifying effect on the body, helping to remove accumulated toxins.

7. **Spiritual Growth:** In Ayurveda and certain spiritual traditions, Sattvic foods are believed to be conducive to spiritual growth and self-awareness. By consuming foods that are considered pure and harmonious, individuals may find it easier to connect with their inner selves.

8. **Reduced Stress:** Sattvic foods are considered to have a calming influence on the nervous system. A Sattvic breakfast may help reduce stress and anxiety, promoting a sense of tranquility.

9. **Environmental Considerations:** Sattvic foods are often plant-based and locally sourced, which can contribute to sustainable and eco-friendly eating habits.

It's important to note that while Sattvic foods have these potential advantages, your individual dietary needs and preferences can vary. What works well for one person may not work the same way for another. If you have special circumstances and health conditions please consult with your health practitioner before adopting a Sattvic diet or incorporating Sattvic meals into your routine. The Sattvic Method is not a substitute for any medical advice, it is however a holistic, alternative method that is based on ancient Hindu Sciences.

Sattvic foods are versatile as they use the seasonally, locally available resources to create their sustainable meal. We need to however get the appropriate spice to detox and clean the body.

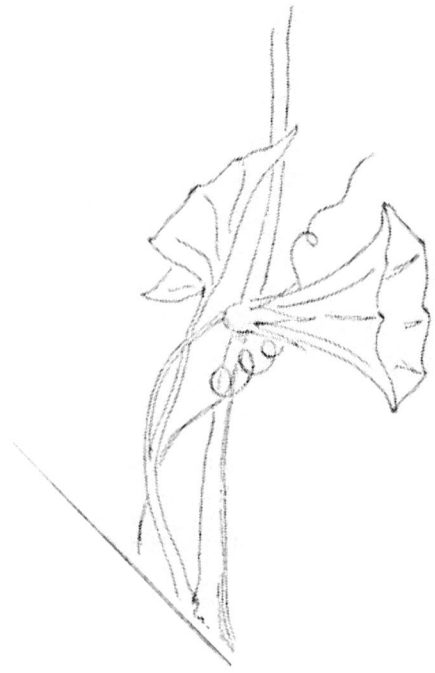

About South Indian Cuisine

Traditional Sattvic South Indian vegetarian cuisine can be considered as nutraceutical due to its focus on holistic well-being and the use of ingredients that have health-promoting properties[1]. Nutraceuticals are foods or food components that provide health benefits beyond basic nutrition, and Sattvic cuisine aligns with this concept in several ways:

1. **Balanced Nutrition:** Sattvic cuisine is well-balanced, providing all essential nutrients required for good health. It includes a variety of whole grains, legumes, vegetables, fruits, nuts, and dairy products, which collectively offer a wide range of vitamins, minerals, and macronutrients like carbohydrates, proteins, and healthy fats.

2. **Herbs and Spices:** South Indian cuisine is known for its use of herbs and spices, such as turmeric, ginger, garlic, and various medicinal herbs like neem and tulsi. Many of these ingredients have potent antioxidant, anti-inflammatory, and antimicrobial properties that contribute to overall health.

3. **Fermented Foods:** Fermented foods like idli, dosa, and yogurt are staples in South Indian cuisine. These foods are rich in probiotics, which support gut health and boost the immune system.

4. **Low in Processed Foods:** Sattvic cuisine tends to be low in processed foods, artificial additives, and preservatives, which are often associated with health risks. Instead, it emphasizes natural, whole ingredients.

---

[1] Parthasarathi, S.K., Hebbani, A.V. & Dharmavaram Desai, P.P. Vegetarian ethnic foods of South India: review on the influence of traditional knowledge. *J. Ethn. Food* **9**, 42 (2022). https://doi.org/10.1186/s42779-022-00156-1

5. **Mindful Eating:** Sattvic cuisine places a strong emphasis on mindful eating. Consuming food in a calm and peaceful environment, without distractions, is believed to enhance digestion and overall well-being.

6. **Energy and Prana:** In Ayurveda and Yoga, Sattvic foods are thought to contain high prana, or life energy. This belief suggests that consuming such foods can have a positive impact on one's mental and spiritual well-being.

7. **Seasonal and Local:** South Indian cuisine is typically prepared using seasonal and locally sourced ingredients. This ensures that the food is fresh and retains its nutritional value.

In recent decades due to urbanization and availability of fast foods, there has been a noticeable shift in the lifestyles and food patterns in South India. These changes include:

1. **Increased Consumption of Processed Foods:** Like many other regions, South India has seen an increase in the consumption of processed and fast foods, which are often high in sugar, salt, unhealthy fats, and additives.

2. **Reduced Traditional Cooking:** Busy lifestyles have led to a decline in traditional home cooking. Many people now rely on convenience foods or eat out more frequently.

3. **Diet Diversification:** South Indians have started to incorporate a wider range of cuisines into their diets, including North Indian, Chinese, and Western foods. While this diversification can be exciting, it may sometimes lead to less emphasis on traditional, nutritionally balanced meals.

4. **Health-Consciousness:** There is a growing awareness of the importance of health and nutrition, leading to a renewed interest in traditional ingredients and cooking methods.

Many people are seeking ways to incorporate the health benefits of Sattvic cuisine into their modern diets.

Traditional Sattvic South Indian vegetarian cuisine can be considered nutraceutical due to its focus on holistic health, balanced nutrition, and the use of ingredients with potential health benefits. However, changing lifestyles and dietary habits in South India have led to some shifts in food patterns, including increased consumption of processed foods. Efforts to balance modern convenience with the nutritional wisdom of traditional cuisine can help promote better health outcomes in both short and long term.

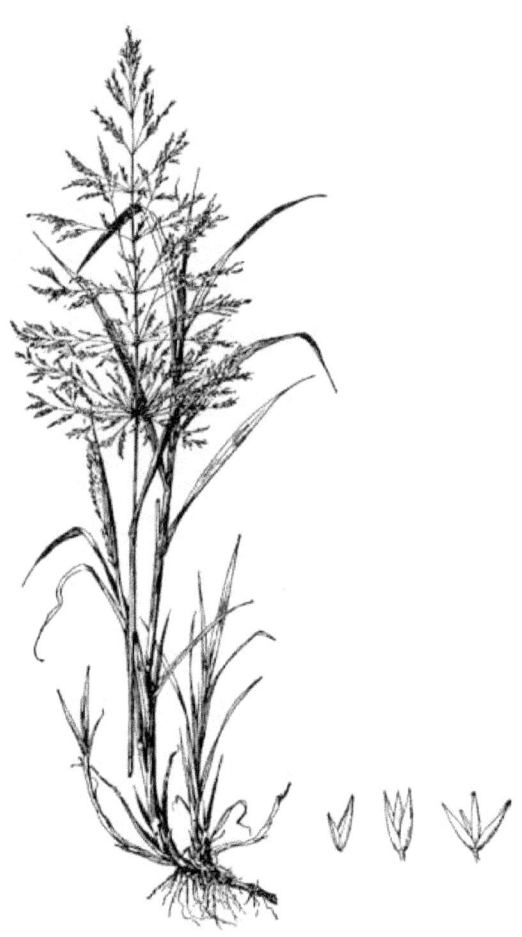

Importance of Preserving Traditional Breakfast

The rate of change in food preferences in South India, as in many other parts of the world, has seen a significant shift from traditional to Westernized dietary patterns. This shift encompasses changes from homemade to ready-made or processed foods[2]. While these changes offer convenience, they also come with several deleterious effects on health:

1. **Increased Consumption of Processed Foods:** Ready-made and processed foods, often high in sugar, unhealthy fats, and artificial additives, have become more readily available and convenient. This has led to an increased consumption of snacks, fast food, and pre-packaged meals.

2. **Rise in Sugar and Salt Intake:** Many processed foods are loaded with added sugars and high levels of salt. Excessive sugar intake is associated with a range of health issues, including obesity, type 2 diabetes, and dental problems. High salt intake can lead to hypertension and cardiovascular diseases.

3. **Trans Fats and Unhealthy Fats:** Some processed foods contain trans fats and unhealthy saturated fats, which are linked to heart disease and other chronic conditions. These fats are often used in fried snacks and fast food items.

4. **Lower Nutrient Density:** Processed foods are generally lower in essential nutrients compared to whole, homemade meals. As a result, people may consume more calories without getting the necessary vitamins, minerals, and fiber, potentially leading to malnutrition and overeating.

---

[2] Omidvar, S., & Begum, K. (2014). Dietary pattern, food habits, and preferences among adolescent and adult student girls from an Urban Area, South India. *Indian Journal of Fundamental and Applied Life Sciences*, *4*(2), 465-473.

5. **Reduced Fiber Intake:** Processed foods are often devoid of dietary fiber, which is crucial for digestive health and preventing conditions like constipation and diverticulitis. High-fiber foods also help control blood sugar levels and promote satiety.

6. **Impact on Gut Health:** Ready-made foods may lack the probiotics found in traditionally fermented South Indian dishes. This can negatively affect gut health, potentially leading to digestive problems and a weakened immune system.

7. **Risk of Foodborne Illnesses:** While homemade meals allow for better control over food safety, ready-made foods may pose a higher risk of foodborne illnesses if not stored or handled properly.

8. **Dependency on Convenience:** The convenience of ready-made foods can lead to a decreased emphasis on cooking and traditional culinary skills. This shift can result in a loss of cultural and familial food traditions.

9. **Negative Impact on Health Outcomes:** The shift towards Westernized diets and processed foods has been linked to a rise in non-communicable diseases in South India, including obesity, diabetes, heart disease, and certain types of cancer.

10. **Environmental Impact:** The production and packaging of processed foods often have a larger environmental footprint due to resource-intensive processes and excessive packaging waste.

Efforts to mitigate the deleterious effects of ready-made foods in South India include:

1. **Nutrition Education:** Promoting nutrition education and awareness about the health risks associated with excessive consumption of processed foods.

2. **Government Regulation:** Implementing regulations and taxation policies to discourage the consumption of unhealthy processed foods and promote healthier alternatives.

3. **Supporting Local and Traditional Food Systems:** Encouraging the consumption of local, seasonal, and traditional foods that are often more nutritious and sustainable.
4. **Promoting Home Cooking:** Encouraging home cooking and teaching culinary skills to maintain traditional food culture and control ingredient quality.
5. **Food Labeling:** Improving food labeling to provide consumers with clearer information about the nutritional content of processed foods.
6. **Community Initiatives:** Supporting community-based initiatives that promote healthy eating habits and access to fresh, local ingredients.

In conclusion, the shift from traditional homemade South Indian cuisine to Westernized, ready-made foods has raised concerns about its impact on health and culture. Addressing these issues requires a multi-faceted approach, including education, regulation, and community efforts, to promote healthier dietary choices and maintain the rich culinary heritage of the region.

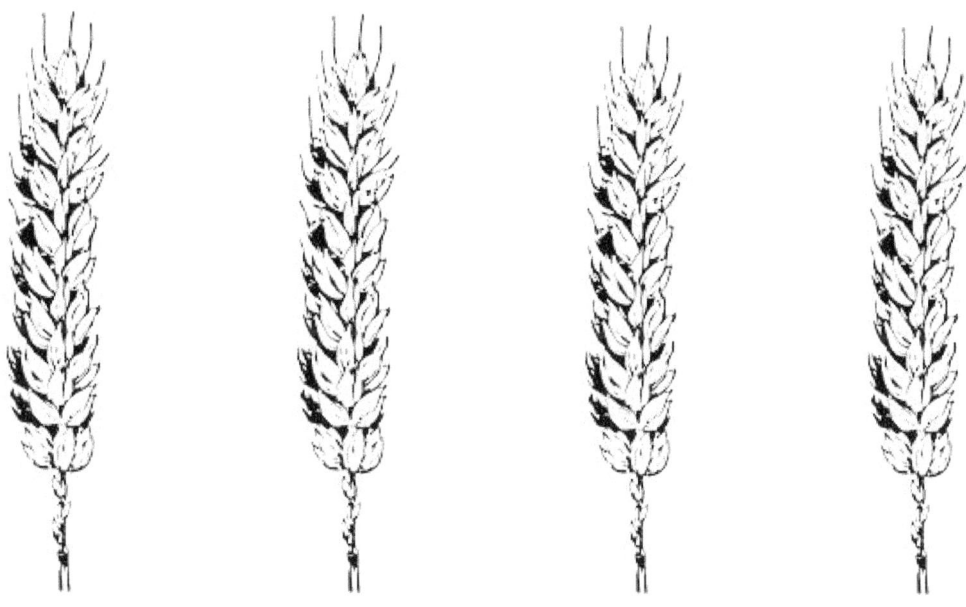

1. Adai

Adai is a South Indian pancake or dosa made from a mixture of different lentils and rice. It's a protein-rich, gluten-free dish and is usually thicker and heavier than regular dosas. Adai is often served with coconut chutney, avial (a mixed vegetable dish), or jaggery for a balanced and satisfying meal. Adai is a nutritious and wholesome dish that's packed with protein and fiber from the lentils. It's a great option for a healthy and filling breakfast or dinner. Enjoy!

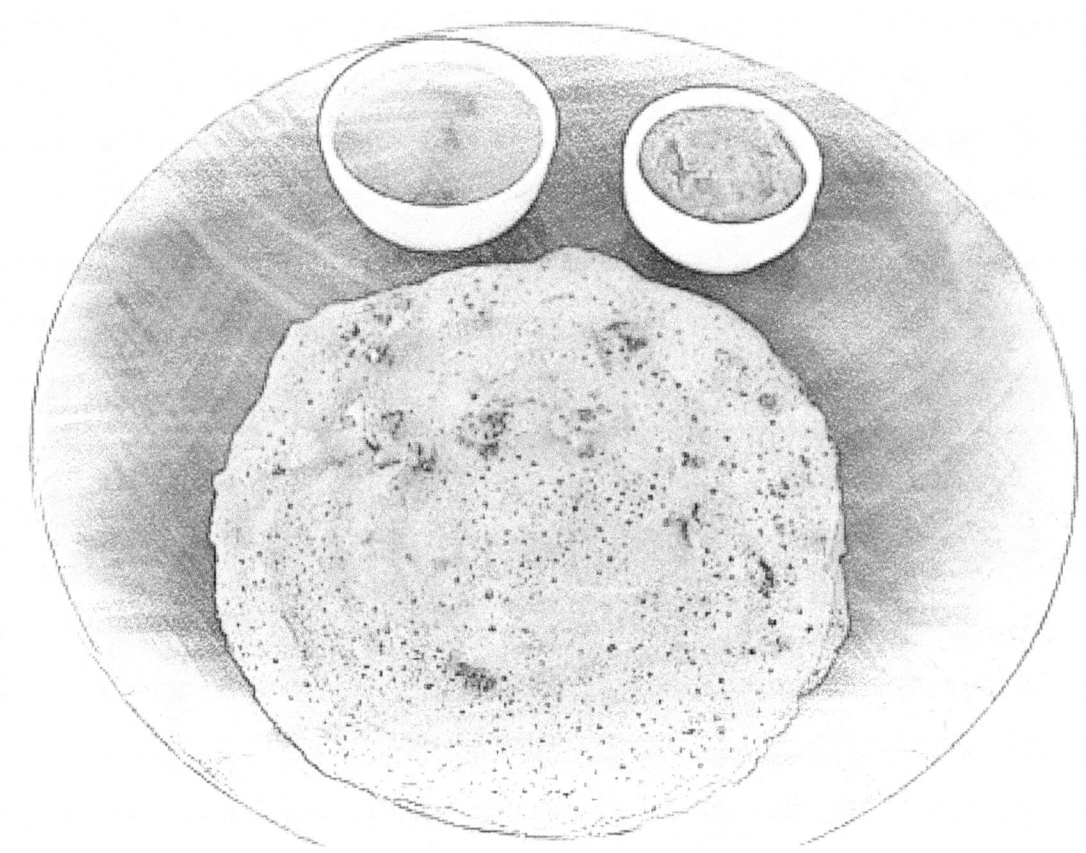

Ingredients:

For the Adai batter:

- 1 cup raw rice
- 1/2 cup parboiled rice (idli rice)
- 1/4 cup split pigeon peas (toor dal)
- 1/4 cup split black gram (urad dal)
- 2 tablespoons Bengal gram (chana dal)
- 2 tablespoons yellow split dal (moong dal)
- 2-3 dried red chilies (adjust to your spice preference)
- 1/2 teaspoon cumin seeds (jeera)
- 1/2 teaspoon black peppercorns (adjust to taste)
- 1/4 teaspoon asafoetida (hing)
- Salt to taste
- Water (for soaking and grinding)

Instructions:

To make Adai batter:

1. Wash the raw rice and parboiled rice together under cold water until the water runs clear. Soak them in enough water for about 4-6 hours or overnight.
2. In a separate bowl, wash and soak the lentils (toor dal, urad dal, chana dal, and moong dal) together for the same duration.
3. Drain the soaked rice and lentils separately.
4. In a blender or food processor, add the soaked rice, red chilies, cumin seeds, black peppercorns, asafoetida, and salt.

5. Add a little water and grind everything into a slightly coarse batter. The batter should have some texture, but it should not be too smooth.

6. Transfer the ground rice mixture to a large mixing bowl.

7. Now, grind the soaked lentils into a smooth paste using a little water.

8. Combine the lentil paste with the ground rice mixture. Mix well to form a thick batter. The consistency should be similar to that of regular dosa batter.

For making Adai:

- 1 green onion, finely chopped (optional)
- 2-3 sprigs of fresh curry leaves, chopped
- 2-3 tablespoons fresh cilantro (coriander leaves), chopped
- Oil or ghee (clarified butter) for cooking

To make Adai:

1. Heat a tava (griddle) or a non-stick pan over medium heat.
2. Grease the tava with a little oil or ghee.
3. Pour a ladleful of the Adai batter onto the hot tava.
4. Using the back of the ladle, gently spread the batter into a thick, round pancake.
5. Sprinkle chopped cabbage or grated carrot, curry leaves, and cilantro on top (if using).
6. Drizzle a few drops of oil or ghee around the edges of the Adai.

7. Cook the Adai on medium heat until the bottom side is golden brown and crispy.

8. Flip the Adai and cook the other side until it's browned and cooked through.

9. Repeat the process with the remaining batter, adding oil or ghee as needed for each Adai.

10. Serve the hot Adai with coconut chutney, aviyal, or jaggery.

Serving Suggestions:

Video of Adai dosai https://youtu.be/bkjdLYnnJTU

Almond-banana pudding https://youtu.be/KB2Vl3Y9uOE

Ginger Cucumber relish https://youtu.be/cvPbFuWJV8E

Aviyal https://youtu.be/Bm9VB0HPg5A

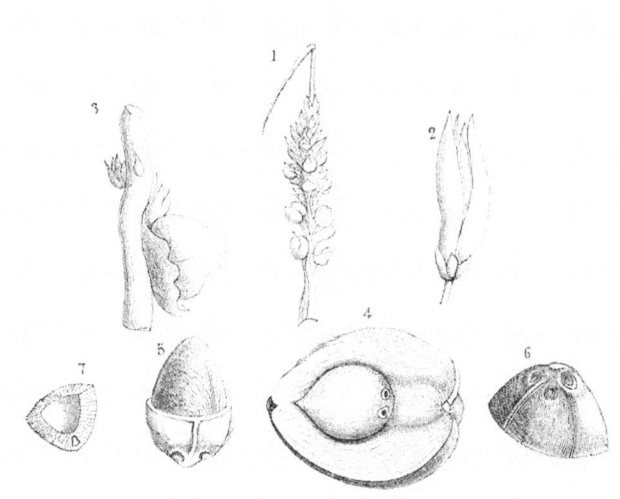

Fig. 190 à 196. — Régime, fleur et fruit du Cocos nucifera L.

2. Akki Roti

Akki Roti is a popular South Indian flatbread made from rice flour and flavored with various spices and vegetables. It's a delicious and gluten-free dish that's often served for breakfast. Akki Roti is best enjoyed fresh off the griddle when it's still warm and crispy. It's a nutritious and flavorful dish that's loved for its simplicity and versatility.

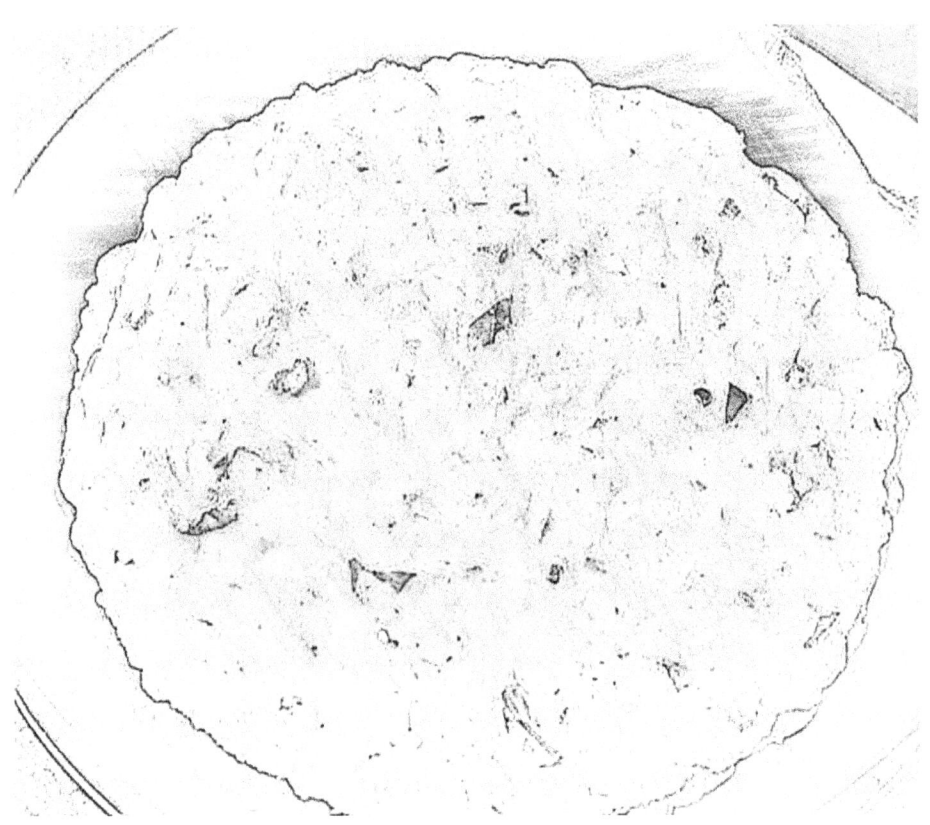

Ingredients:

For Making Dough:

- 1 cup rice flour
- 1/4 cup finely grated fresh coconut (optional)
- 1/2 cup finely chopped mixed vegetables (carrots, red chilies, cilantro, etc.)
-
- 2-3 tablespoons finely chopped fresh cilantro (coriander leaves)
- 1 teaspoon cumin seeds (jeera)
- Salt to taste
- Water (for kneading)
- Oil or ghee (clarified butter) for cooking

Instructions:

1. **Prepare the Dough:**
    - In a mixing bowl, combine the rice flour, grated coconut (if using), chopped vegetables, fresh cilantro, cumin seeds, and salt to taste.
    - Gradually add water, a little at a time, and knead the mixture into a soft, pliable dough. The amount of water needed may vary, so add it slowly until you achieve the right consistency.
    - The dough should be firm enough to hold together but soft enough to roll out easily.

2. **Shape the Rotis:**
    - Divide the dough into equal portions, roughly the size of a lemon.

- Take one portion of the dough and flatten it with your fingers on a clean, dry surface. Alternatively, you can use a plastic sheet or banana leaf for easy handling.
- Shape it into a round or oval roti, about 1/4 to 1/2 inch thick. You can use your fingers or a rolling pin for this.

3. **Cook the Rotis:**
    - Heat a tava (griddle) or a non-stick pan over medium heat.
    - Once the tava is hot, place the shaped roti gently on it.
    - Drizzle a little oil or ghee around the edges of the roti and a little in the center as well.
    - Cook the roti for about 2-3 minutes on one side until it's lightly browned.
    - Flip the roti and cook the other side for another 2-3 minutes until it's golden brown and crisp.
    - Press the edges gently with a spatula to ensure even cooking.
    - Remove the Akki Roti from the tava and serve hot.

Serving suggestions:

Video version of a simple recipe for Akki roti https://youtu.be/2YhkstkJrYU

Sattvic Eggplant Saung https://youtu.be/9sCR3K0Eq3U

Potato Eriyal https://youtu.be/lm7A7pmILGU

3. Aapam

Aapam is a popular South Indian pancake that's soft in the center with a thin, crispy edge. It's made from fermented rice and coconut batter. Aapam is a delightful South Indian dish that's both healthy and delicious. Its unique texture and mild coconut flavor make it a great addition to any meal. Enjoy!

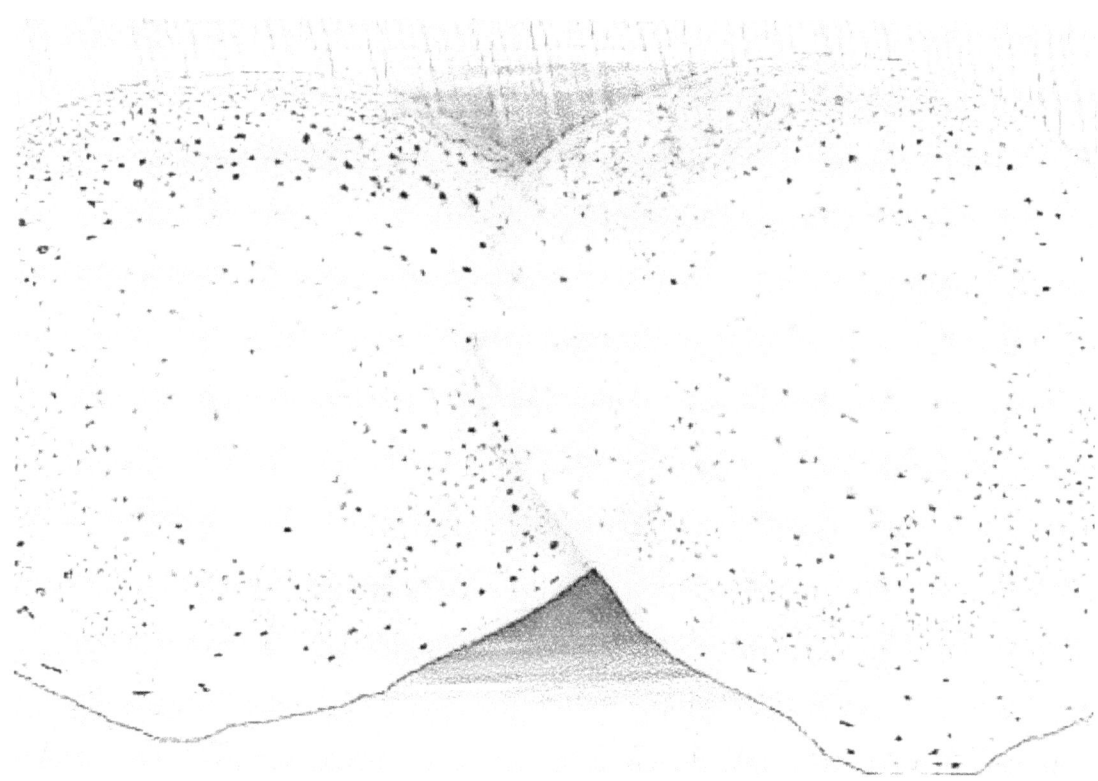

Ingredients:

For the Batter:

- 1 cup raw rice (sona masuri or any short-grain variety)
- 1/4 cup cooked rice
- 1/4 cup grated fresh coconut
- 1/2 teaspoon active dry yeast or 1 teaspoon instant yeast
- 1/2 teaspoon sugar
- 1/2 cup lukewarm water (for dissolving yeast)
- 1/4 teaspoon salt (adjust to taste)

Instructions:

For Making the Batter:

1. Wash the raw rice thoroughly in cold water until the water runs clear. Soak the rice in enough water for 4-6 hours or overnight.
2. In a separate bowl, dissolve the yeast and sugar in lukewarm water. Let it sit for about 10-15 minutes until it becomes frothy.
3. Drain the soaked rice and add it to a blender.
4. Add the cooked rice, grated coconut, and a pinch of salt to the blender.
5. Pour the yeast mixture into the blender as well.
6. Blend everything together until you get a smooth batter. The batter should be of pouring consistency, similar to dosa batter. You can add a little water if it's too thick.
7. Transfer the batter to a large bowl.

8. Cover the bowl with a lid or a clean cloth and let it ferment in a warm place for 6-8 hours or overnight. The fermentation time may vary depending on the temperature in your kitchen. The batter should double in volume and become slightly bubbly.

You need for cooking Aapam:

- 1 teaspoon oil or ghee (clarified butter) per aapam
- A non-stick aapam pan (aapachatti)

Instructions for Making Aapam:

1. After the fermentation period, check the batter. It should be airy and slightly bubbly. If it's too thick, you can add a little water to adjust the consistency.
2. Heat the aapam pan (appachatti) over medium-high heat. Brush it with a little oil or ghee to grease it.
3. Pour a ladleful of batter into the center of the pan.
4. Hold the handles of the pan and gently swirl it in a circular motion to spread the batter thinly and evenly, creating a lace-like pattern around the edges. You can tilt the pan slightly to ensure that the batter forms a thin layer.
5. Cover the pan with a lid and let the aapam cook over medium heat for about 2-3 minutes. The edges should turn crispy, and the center should be soft.

6. Once the aapam is cooked, remove it from the pan using a spatula. It should come off easily because of the non-stick surface.

7. Repeat the process with the remaining batter, greasing the pan lightly before making each aapam.

8. Serve the aapams hot with your favorite accompaniment, such as coconut milk, stew, or a spicy curry.

Serving suggestions:

Potato saagu https://youtu.be/jlQ8FMdr7dA

Moong dal chutney https://youtu.be/6D1lkA1i-tU

Molagapodi https://youtu.be/yyN9cssAoZo

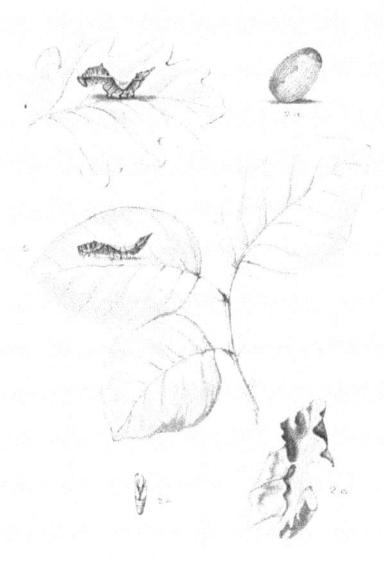

4. Atho

This dish has its origins in Burma, whose Tamil refugees make for a fascinating story in itself. It's a mixture of spicy noodles, shredded cabbage and onions seasoned with salt, tamarind, chilli flakes and garlic. This recipe excludes onions and garlic and has added some ginger. Atho, also known as Burmese Atho, is a popular street food in Myanmar (Burma). It's a flavorful and spicy salad made with flat rice noodles, various ingredients, and a special chili sauce.

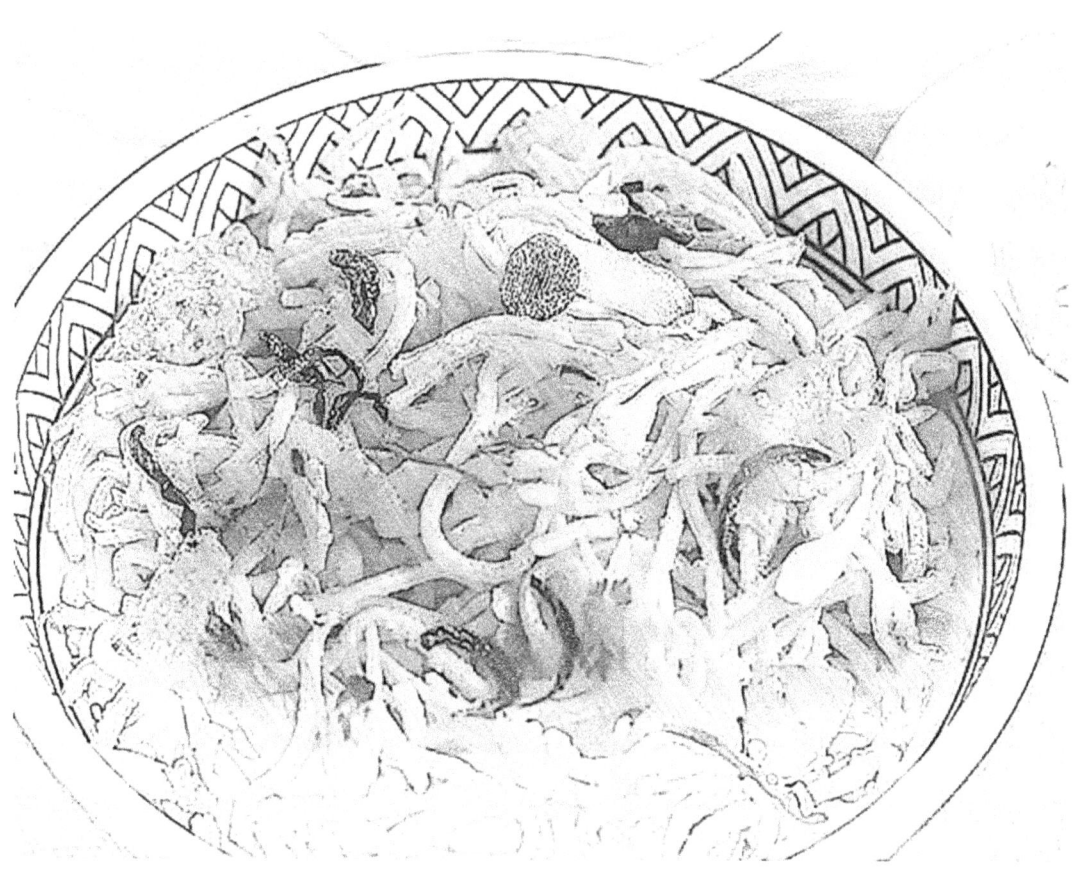

Ingredients:

For Making the Noodles:

- 200 grams flat rice noodles (thin variety)
- Water for boiling
- 1/2 teaspoon salt
- Ice water (for soaking)

Instructions:

Prepare the Noodles:

1. Bring a large pot of water to a boil. Add a pinch of salt.
2. Add the flat rice noodles to the boiling water and cook for about 2-3 minutes or until they are soft but still have some texture (al dente).
3. Drain the noodles and immediately transfer them to a bowl of ice water to stop the cooking process. This also helps to separate the noodles and keep them from sticking together.
4. Once cooled, drain the noodles thoroughly and set them aside.

Next make the chili sauce fresh to give your recipe the best taste and assemble it together. Follow the instructions below.

You need for the Chili Sauce:

- 4-5 dried red chilies
- 1 teaspoon sugar
- 1 teaspoon miso sauce (optional)
- 1 teaspoon doenjang (optional)
- Juice of 1 lime or lemon
- Salt to taste

Make the Chili Sauce:

1. Soak the dried red chilies in warm water for about 15-20 minutes to soften them.
2. Drain the chilies and remove the seeds if you prefer a milder sauce.
3. In a mortar and pestle or a blender, combine the soaked chilies, shallot (if using), miso paste (if using), doenjang (if using), sugar, lime or lemon juice, and a pinch of salt.
4. Pound or blend everything into a smooth paste. Adjust the seasoning to your taste by adding more sugar, salt, or lime juice if needed.

You need for the Toppings:

- 1/4 cup cabbage, finely shredded
- 1/4 cup carrot, julienned
- 1/4 cup cucumber, julienned
- 1/4 cup red papaya, julienned (optional)
- 1/4 cup fried chickpea fritters (optional)
- Roasted peanuts, crushed (optional)
- Fresh cilantro leaves
- Lime or lemon wedges

To assemble the Atho:

1. In a large mixing bowl, combine the cooked and drained rice noodles with the shredded cabbage, julienned carrot, cucumber, red papaya (if using), and any other toppings you like.
2. Pour the chili sauce over the ingredients in the bowl.
3. Toss everything together until the noodles and vegetables are coated with the sauce.
4. Serve the Atho garnished with fried chickpea fritters, crushed roasted peanuts, fresh cilantro leaves, and lime or lemon wedges on the side.
5. Atho can be enjoyed as a spicy and tangy salad.

Serving suggestions

Aama vada https://youtu.be/sJ3tfA1dJ4Q

Cabbage pakoda https://youtu.be/vY4jSb13fGI

Bonda https://youtu.be/N5NvBE-RSgI

5. Aval Upma

Aval, also known as poha (in Hindi) or flattened rice, is a versatile ingredient in Indian cuisine.

It's often used to make a variety of dishes, including breakfast options, snacks, and even desserts.

Aval Upma is a quick and delicious dish that can be customized with your favorite vegetables

and spices.

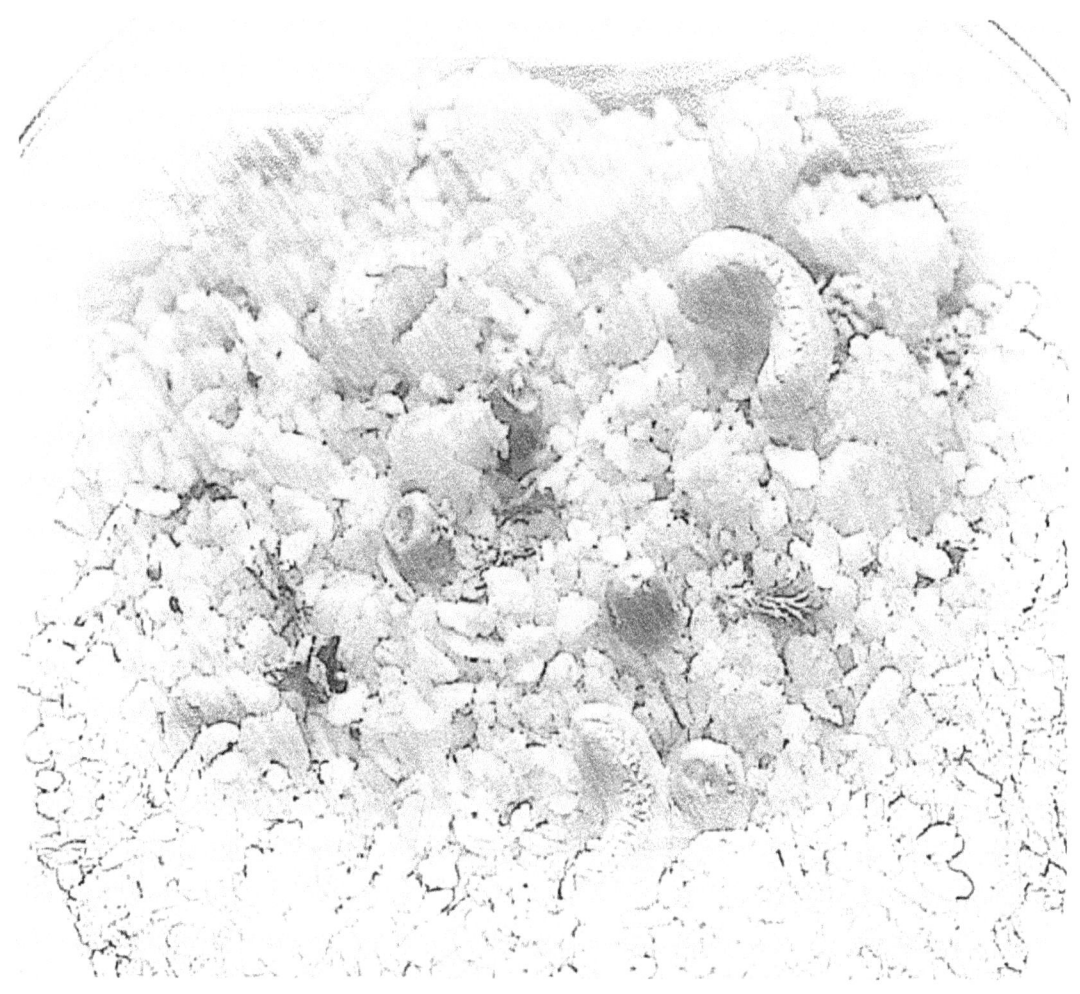

Ingredients:

- 1 cup thick aval (poha/flattened rice)
- 2 tablespoons oil
- 1/2 teaspoon mustard seeds
- 1 tablespoon cashew nut
- 1/2 teaspoon urad dal (split black gram)
- 1/2 teaspoon chana dal (split chickpeas)
- 1-2 red chilies, chopped (adjust to your spice preference)
- A pinch of asafoetida (hing)
- 1/2 teaspoon turmeric powder
- 1 bunch green onion, chopped
- ¼ cup green peas
- A few curry leaves
- Salt to taste
- Fresh coriander leaves for garnish (optional)
- Lemon juice (optional, for tanginess)

Instructions:

1. Place the aval in a sieve or colander and rinse it under running water for a few seconds. Gently fluff the aval with your fingers as you rinse it. Drain well and set it aside.
2. Heat oil in a pan or kadai over medium heat.
3. Add mustard seeds and let them splutter.
4. Add cashew nut, urad dal, and chana dal. Sauté until they turn golden brown.
5. Add chopped red chilies and a pinch of asafoetida. Sauté for a minute until the chilies become slightly soft.
6. Add curry leaves and chopped red onions. Sauté until the red onions turn translucent.
7. Add chopped tomatoes and cook until they become soft and mushy.

8. Add turmeric powder and mix well.
9. Add the rinsed and drained aval to the pan. Mix everything together gently, ensuring the aval is well coated with the spices.
10. Add salt to taste and mix again.
11. Reduce the heat to low, cover the pan with a lid, and let the aval cook for about 5 minutes. There's no need to add water as the aval will absorb the moisture from the steam.
12. After 5 minutes, remove the lid and gently fluff the aval with a fork.
13. If you like, you can squeeze some fresh lemon juice over the Aval Upma for a tangy flavor.
14. Garnish with fresh coriander leaves if desired.
15. Serve the Aval Upma hot as a breakfast dish.

Serving suggestions:

This video shows how to make a version of Aval https://youtu.be/UeMTRcyz6MA

Chickpea stew https://youtu.be/dnxs3xQpf6U

Delicious Red Soup https://youtu.be/y8pxazCTLy0

Raita https://youtu.be/Svd7w-MsLd8

6. Bisi Bele Baath

Bisi Bele Baath is a flavorful and wholesome South Indian rice dish made with rice, lentils, and a medley of vegetables. The name "Bisi Bele Bath" translates to "hot lentil rice" in Kannada, reflecting its slightly spicy and aromatic nature. Bisi Bele Bath is a delightful and wholesome dish that's rich in flavors and textures. Enjoy it as a comforting one-pot meal.

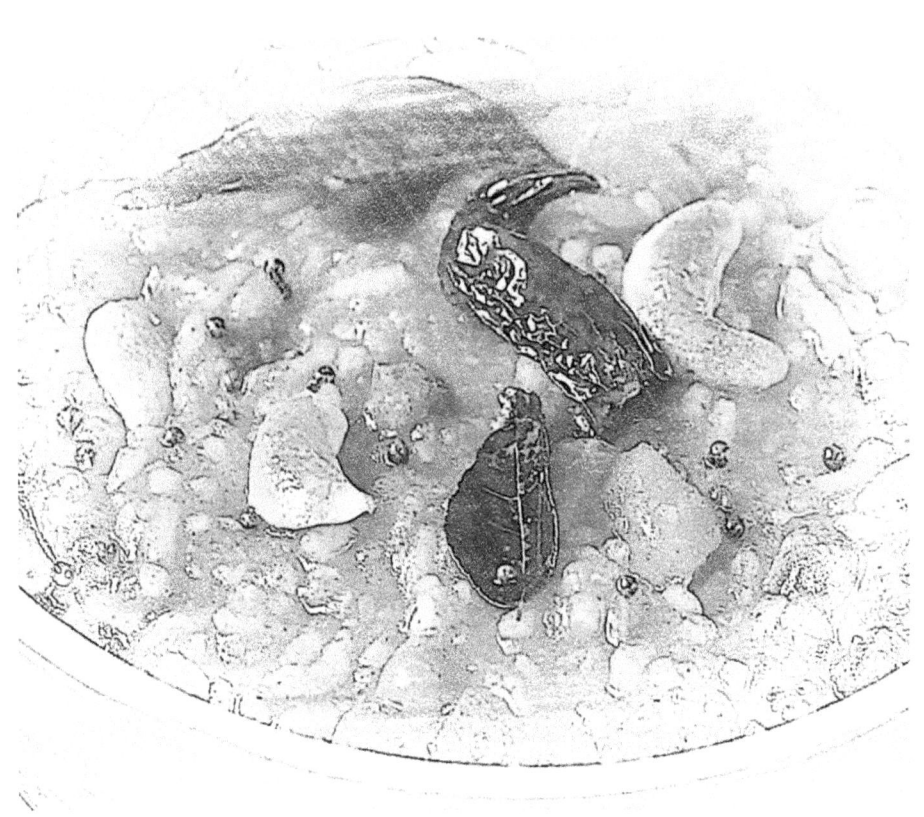

Ingredients:

For the Spice Powder:

- 2 tablespoons coriander seeds
- 1 tablespoon chana dal (split chickpeas)
- 1/2 tablespoon urad dal (split black gram)
- 1/2 teaspoon fenugreek seeds (methi seeds)
- 4-5 dried red chilies (adjust to your spice preference)
- 1/2 teaspoon cumin seeds (jeera)
- 1/4 teaspoon black peppercorns
- 1/4 teaspoon asafoetida (hing)

Instructions:

To make the Spice Powder:

1. Heat a dry pan over medium heat and add all the spice powder ingredients except asafoetida.
2. Roast them until they become aromatic and the dals turn golden brown. Be careful not to burn them.
3. Add asafoetida and roast for another 30 seconds. Remove from heat and let the spices cool.
4. Once cooled, grind them into a fine powder using a spice grinder or mortar and pestle. This spice powder is the key to the unique flavor of Bisi Bele Baath.

Ingredients:

You need for the Bisi Bele Baath:

- 1 cup rice (any variety)
- 1/2 cup toor dal (split pigeon peas)
- 1/2 cup mixed vegetables (carrots, beans, peas, etc.), chopped
- 1 small tomato, chopped
- 2 tablespoons tamarind pulp (soak a small piece of tamarind in warm water and extract the pulp)
- 2 tablespoons ghee (clarified butter) or oil
- 1/2 teaspoon mustard seeds
- A pinch of asafoetida (hing)
- 10-12 curry leaves
- 2 tablespoons roasted peanuts
- 2 tablespoons grated coconut (fresh or frozen)
- Salt to taste
- Water (for cooking rice and dal)
- Chopped coriander leaves for garnish (optional)

Instruction:

For the Rice and Lentils:

1. Rinse the rice and toor dal separately under cold water until the water runs clear.
2. In a large saucepan, combine the rinsed rice and toor dal. Add 4 cups of water and cook them together until they are soft and well-cooked. You can use a pressure cooker for faster cooking. Once cooked, set them aside.

For the Bisi Bele Baath:

1. Heat ghee or oil in a large, heavy-bottomed pot over medium heat.
2. Add mustard seeds and let them splutter.
3. Add asafoetida and curry leaves. Sauté for a few seconds.
4. Add chopped onions and sauté until they turn translucent.
5. Add chopped tomatoes and cook until they become soft and mushy.
6. Add the mixed vegetables and cook for a few minutes until they start to soften.
7. Add the tamarind pulp and the ground spice powder. Mix well and cook for a couple of minutes.
8. Add salt to taste and mix.
9. Add the cooked rice and dal mixture to the pot. Mix everything together.
10. Add 2-3 cups of water to achieve the desired consistency. Bisi Bele Bath should have a semi-thick, porridge-like consistency. Adjust the water accordingly.
11. Let the Bisi Bele Baath simmer over low heat for about 10-15 minutes, allowing the flavors to meld together.
12. In a separate pan, roast the peanuts until they are golden brown.
13. Add roasted peanuts and grated coconut to the Bisi Bele Baath. Mix well.
14. Taste and adjust salt and spice levels as needed.

Serve Bisi Bele Baath:

1. Garnish with chopped coriander leaves (if using).
2. Serve Bisi Bele Baath hot with ghee, fried chips etc.

Serving Suggestions:

Lentil Patties https://youtu.be/1Uyf0WwYbZE

Ghee https://youtu.be/s6hL61F5BSQ

Bittermelon chips https://youtu.be/HLcpnDFwdVc

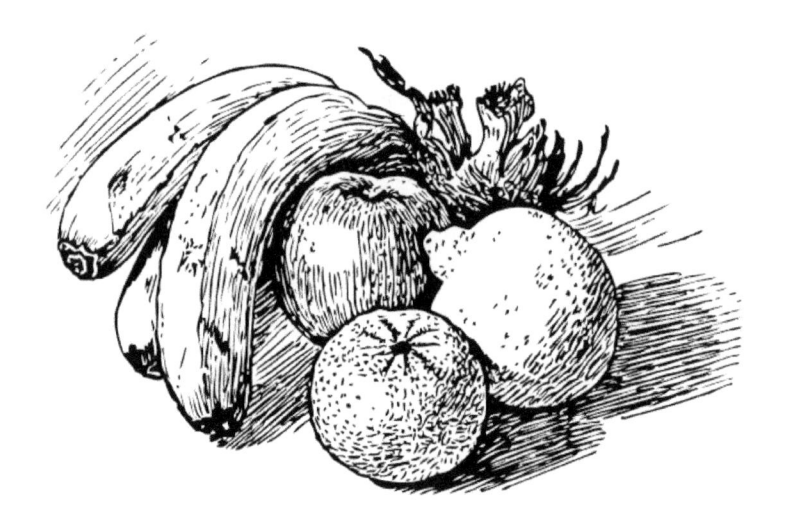

7. Chana Sundal

Chana Sundal is a sattvic and healthy South Indian snack or side dish made from chickpeas (chana) and flavored with coconut and mild spices. It's often prepared during festivals and as an offering to deities in South Indian households. Chana Sundal is not only nutritious but also delicious with its blend of flavors and textures. Enjoy it as a healthy and sattvic addition to your meals.

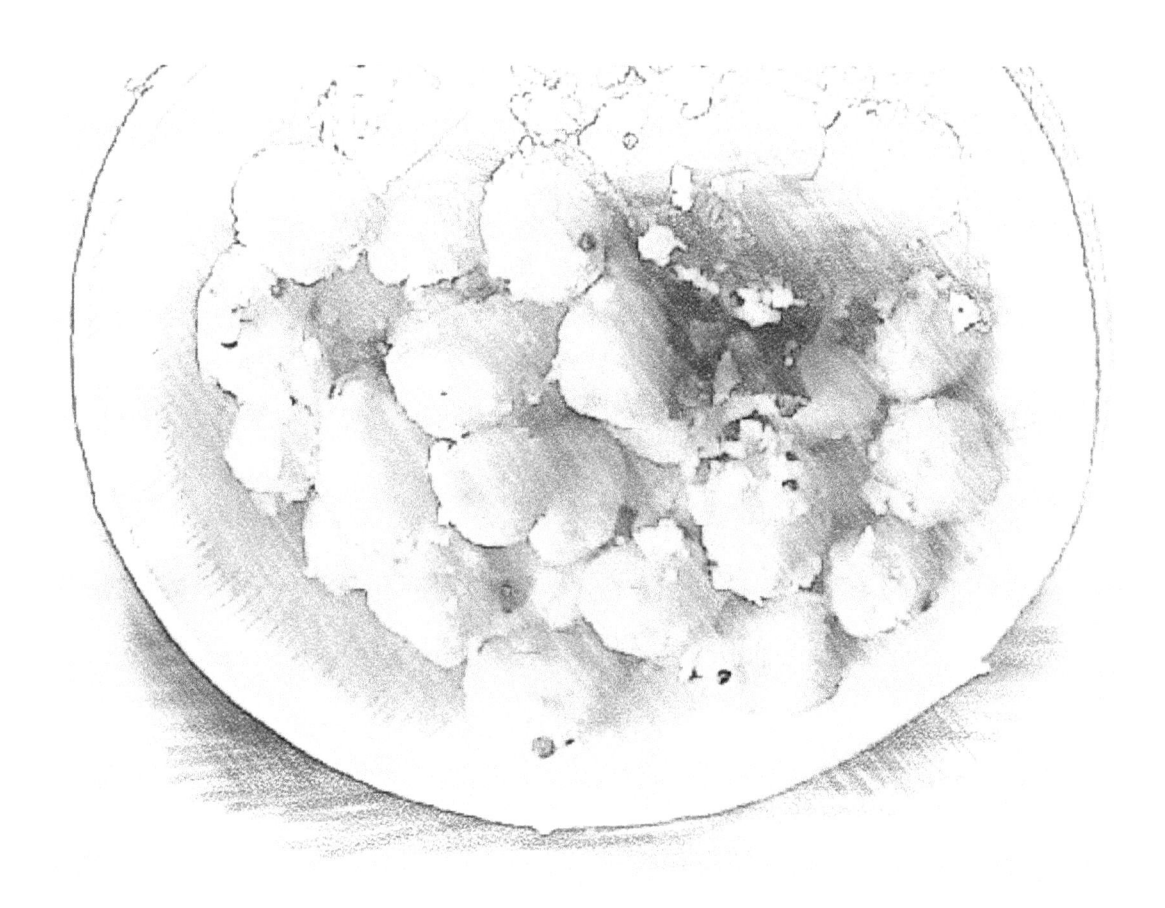

Ingredients:

- 1 cup dried chickpeas (kabuli chana), soaked overnight
- 2 tablespoons grated coconut (fresh or frozen)
- 1-2 red chilies, finely chopped (adjust to your spice preference)
- A pinch of asafoetida (hing)
- 1/2 teaspoon mustard seeds
- 1/2 teaspoon urad dal (split black gram)
- A few curry leaves
- 1-2 tablespoons oil (preferably coconut oil)
- Salt to taste
- Fresh coriander leaves for garnish (optional)

Instructions:

To cook the Chickpeas:

1. Drain the soaked chickpeas and rinse them thoroughly.
2. In a large pot, add the soaked chickpeas and enough water to cover them. Add a pinch of salt.
3. Bring the chickpeas to a boil and then reduce the heat to a simmer. Cook for about 30-40 minutes or until the chickpeas are tender but still have a slight bite (al dente). You can also use a pressure cooker to cook them, which will be faster.
4. Once cooked, drain the chickpeas and set them aside.

To make Chana Sundal:

1. Heat oil in a pan over medium heat. Add mustard seeds and let them splutter.

2. Add urad dal and sauté until it turns golden brown.

3. Add a pinch of asafoetida and chopped red chilies. Sauté for a minute until the chilies become slightly soft.

4. Add curry leaves and mix well.

5. Add the cooked chickpeas to the pan and stir to combine with the spices.

6. Season with salt to taste and cook for another 2-3 minutes, allowing the chickpeas to absorb the flavors.

7. Finally, add the grated coconut and toss everything together. Cook for another minute to heat the coconut through. Remove from heat.

Garnish and Serve:

1. Garnish the Chana Sundal with fresh coriander leaves (if using).
2. Serve the Chana Sundal as a sattvic snack or side dish.

Serving Suggestion:

Dosa https://youtu.be/hmueE_40RdU

Sattvic Upma https://youtu.be/IB3i_O37K60

Sattvic bean salad https://youtu.be/j17KbzH27ns

8. Coconut Rice

Coconut rice is a flavorful South Indian dish made with cooked rice, freshly grated coconut, and a blend of aromatic spices. It's a delicious and quick dish that can be served as a main course or as a side dish. Coconut rice is a fragrant and delightful dish that pairs well with a variety of side dishes.

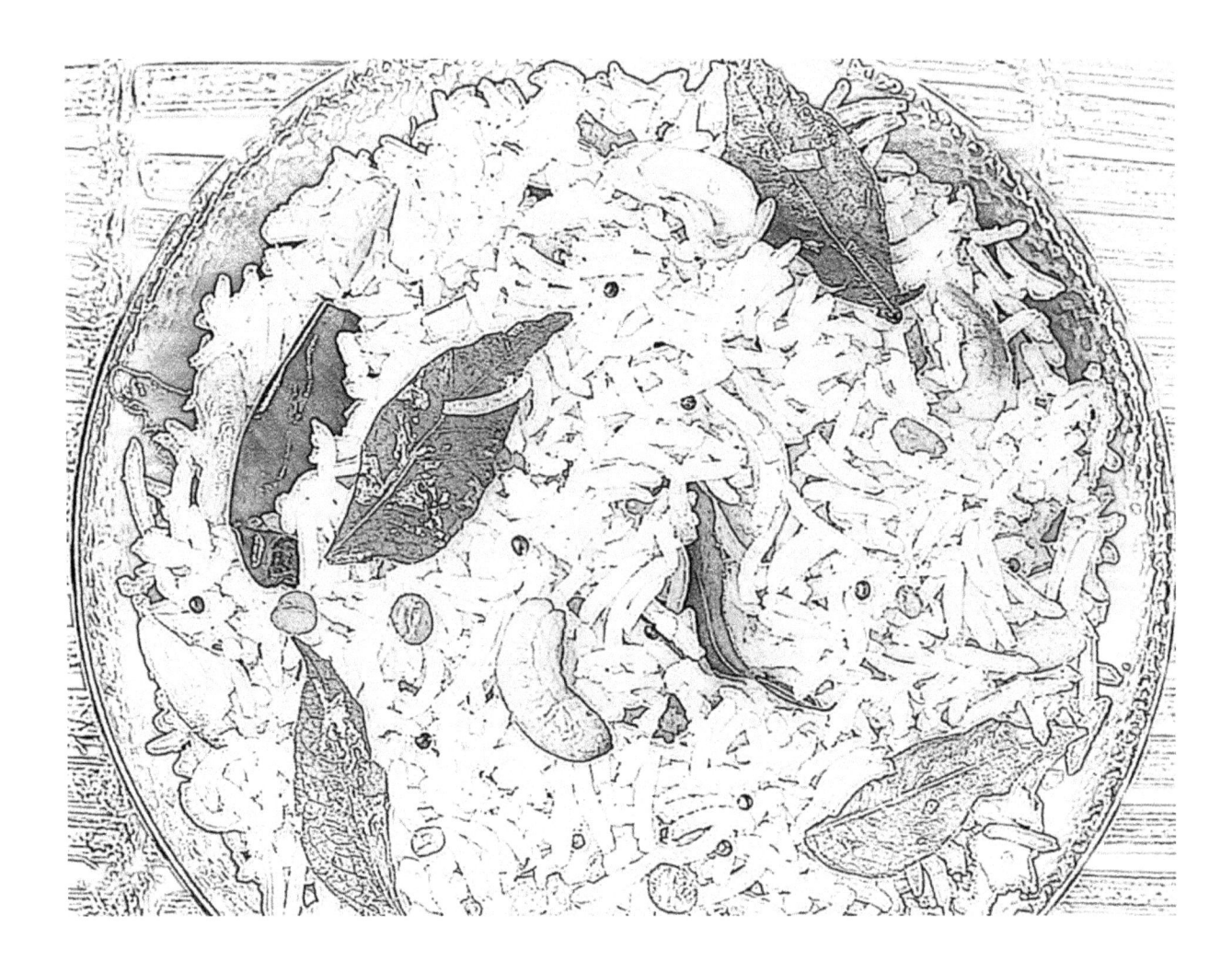

You need:

- 1 cup basmati rice or long-grain rice
- 2 cups water (for cooking rice)
- 1 cup freshly grated coconut
- 2 tablespoons oil or ghee (clarified butter)
- 1/2 teaspoon mustard seeds
- 1/2 teaspoon urad dal (split black gram)
- 1/2 teaspoon chana dal (split chickpeas)
- A pinch of asafoetida (hing)
- 2-3 red chilies, slit lengthwise (adjust to your spice preference)
- 10-12 curry leaves
- 1/4 cup roasted peanuts
- Salt to taste

Instructions:

For cooking the Rice:

1. Rinse the rice thoroughly under cold water until the water runs clear.
2. In a saucepan, combine the rinsed rice and 2 cups of water. Add a pinch of salt and bring it to a boil.
3. Once it comes to a boil, reduce the heat to low, cover the saucepan with a lid, and let the rice simmer for 15-20 minutes or until it's cooked and the grains are separate.
4. Once the rice is cooked, remove it from heat, fluff it with a fork, and let it cool.

For assembling Coconut Rice:

1. Heat oil or ghee in a large pan or kadai over medium heat.

2. Add mustard seeds and let them splutter.
3. Add urad dal and chana dal. Sauté until they turn golden brown.
4. Add a pinch of asafoetida, slit red chilies, and curry leaves. Sauté for a minute until the chilies become slightly soft.
5. Add the freshly grated coconut to the pan and sauté for 2-3 minutes. You can roast it until it turns slightly golden, but make sure it doesn't get overly browned.
6. Add the roasted peanuts and mix well.
7. Now, add the cooked and cooled rice to the pan.
8. Gently mix the rice with the coconut and spice mixture until everything is well combined. Be gentle to avoid breaking the rice grains.
9. Adjust salt to taste and continue to cook for another 2-3 minutes to heat the rice through.
10. Remove from heat and serve hot.

Serving Suggestions:

Serve coconut rice with

Instant Apple Pickle https://youtu.be/kwH-X7zUiXg

Carrot Chutney https://youtu.be/gtBSNX51YPg

Cabbage Sabzi https://youtu.be/3JANBXUf-Hc

9. Dosa

Dosa is a popular South Indian dish made from fermented rice and urad dal (black gram) batter. It's a thin, crispy crepe that's commonly served for breakfast but can also be enjoyed at any time of the day. Dosas are a delightful South Indian delicacy known for their crispness and versatility. Enjoy them for breakfast, lunch, or dinner with your favorite side dishes.

Ingredients:

For the Dosa Batter:

- 1 cup long-grain parboiled rice (Idli rice) or regular rice
- 1/4 cup urad dal (split black gram)
- 1/4 teaspoon fenugreek seeds (methi seeds)
- Salt to taste
- Water (for grinding)

Instructions:

To make Dosa Batter:

1. Wash the rice and urad dal together in cold water until the water runs clear.
2. Soak the washed rice, urad dal, and fenugreek seeds in enough water for about 4-6 hours or overnight.
3. Drain the soaked rice and dal mixture.
4. Add the drained rice and dal mixture to a blender or food processor.
5. Add about 1/2 to 3/4 cup of water and blend into a smooth batter. The batter should have a texture similar to that of pancake batter.
6. Pour the batter into a large mixing bowl.
7. Add salt to taste and mix well.
8. Cover the bowl with a clean cloth or plastic wrap and let it ferment in a warm place for 8-12 hours or until it has doubled in volume. The fermentation time may vary depending on the temperature of your surroundings.

To make Dosas:

1. Heat a non-stick dosa tava (griddle) or a flat frying pan over medium heat.
2. Once the tava is hot, reduce the heat to medium-low and lightly grease it with a few drops of oil or ghee. Pour a ladleful of dosa batter onto the center of the hot tava.
3. Quickly spread the batter in a circular motion to form a thin dosa. The dosa should be thin and crispy.
4. Drizzle a little oil or ghee around the edges of the dosa and a little on top.
5. Cook the dosa until it turns golden brown and crispy on the bottom.
6. Carefully flip the dosa using a spatula and cook the other side until it's golden brown as well.
7. Remove the dosa from the tava and place it on a plate.
8. Repeat the process for the remaining batter, adjusting the heat and greasing the tava as needed.
9. Serve dosas hot with your choice of accompaniments like coconut chutney, sambar, or potato masala.

Serving suggestions:

Molagapodi https://youtu.be/yyN9cssAoZo

Peanut chutney https://youtu.be/T84w1rluU20

Poricha Kuzhambhu https://youtu.be/6D2AWP6STQo

10. Idiyappam

Idiyappam, also known as string hoppers, is a traditional South Indian dish made from rice flour. It's a versatile dish that can be served with various accompaniments like coconut milk, kurma, or vegetable stew. Idiyappam is a delicious and gluten-free dish that's light and easy to digest. You need Idiyappam press (also known as a sev press or sevai maker), Idli steamer or a steamer with perforated plates, and Banana leaves or greased idli plates (for steaming).

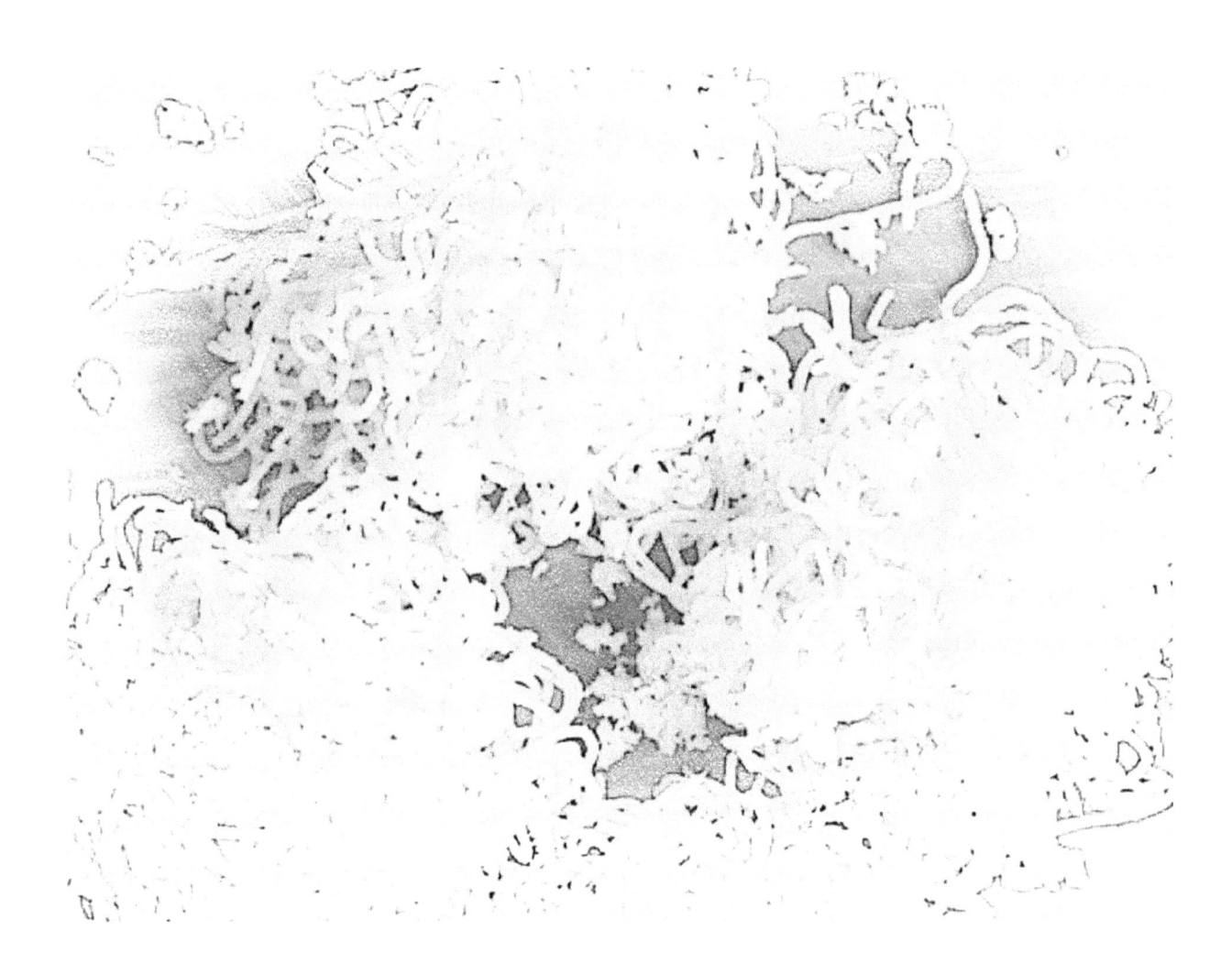

Ingredients:

For the Idiyappam Dough:

- 1 cup rice flour
- 1 cup water
- A pinch of salt
- 1 teaspoon oil

Instructions:

For the Idiyappam Dough:

1. Boil 1 cup of water in a saucepan and add the oil, and a pinch of salt to it.
2. Once the water is boiling, reduce the heat to low and add the rice flour to the hot water.
3. Stir the mixture continuously with a wooden spatula. Ensure that there are no lumps and the rice flour is well combined with the water.
4. Cook the mixture on low heat for about 2-3 minutes. It should come together as a smooth dough. Turn off the heat.
5. Allow the dough to cool for a few minutes until it's warm enough to handle.

To make Idiyappam:

1. Grease the perforated plates of your idli steamer with a little oil or place banana leaves over them.
2. Fill the Idiyappam press with the prepared dough. Make sure to use the plate with small round holes in the press.

3. Press the dough through the holes onto the greased idli plates or banana leaves in a circular, spiral motion to form a round shape. You can also make individual portions.
4. Steam the Idiyappam in an idli steamer or any steamer for about 8-10 minutes or until they are cooked through. They should look firm and glossy when done.
5. Remove the Idiyappam from the steamer and let them cool slightly for a minute or two.
6. Gently transfer them to a serving plate using a flat spatula.

Serving Idiyappam:

1. Idiyappam can be served with a variety of accompaniments. Here are a few options:
   - **Coconut Milk:** You can serve Idiyappam with fresh coconut milk sweetened with a little sugar for a sweet version or salted for a savory version.
   - **Vegetable Stew:** Idiyappam pairs beautifully with vegetable stew, a mild and flavorful coconut-based curry.
   - **Kurma:** You can also serve Idiyappam with a vegetable kurma or any spicy curry of your choice.

Serving Suggestions

Parsley Chutney https://youtu.be/ADth8ETWRR8

Potato Saagu https://youtu.be/jlQ8FMdr7dA

Sattvic Raita https://youtu.be/Svd7w-MsLd8

11. Karuveppilai Rice

Karuveppilai Rice, also known as Curry Leaf Rice, is a flavorful and aromatic South Indian dish that is often considered sattvic because of its use of natural, plant-based ingredients. It's made using fresh curry leaves, rice, and a few spices. Sattvic Karuveppilai Rice is a delicious and aromatic dish that's perfect for a sattvic diet. It's both nutritious and flavorful, making it a wonderful addition to your meal. If you want to make a variation to this recipe to make karuveppilai powder and store it for longer time https://youtu.be/zv0BW1fr-3A

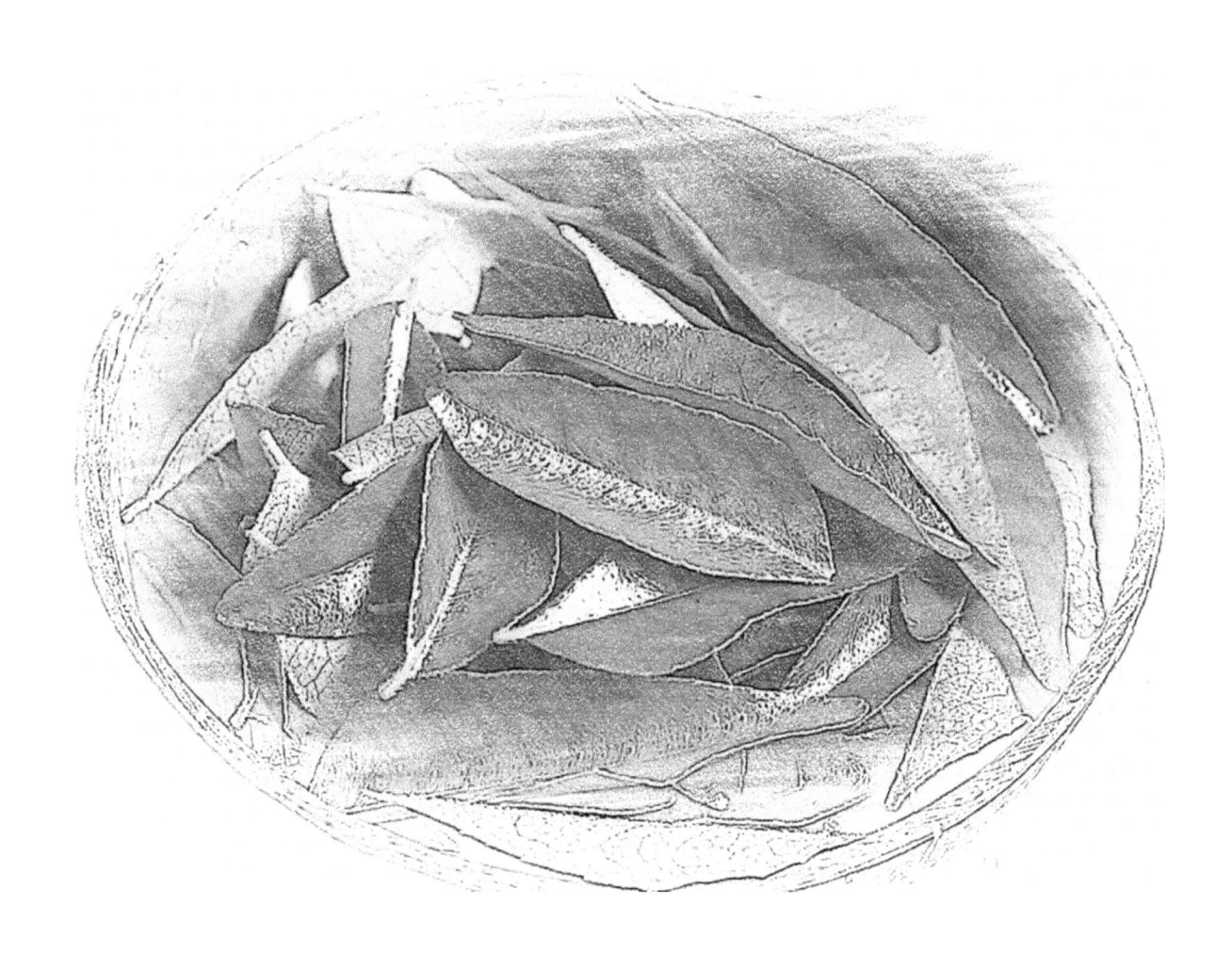

Ingredients:

For making the Rice:

- 1 cup long-grain rice
- 2 cups water (for cooking rice)
- ½ teaspoon oil
- A pinch of salt

Instructions:

To cook Rice:

1. Rinse the rice thoroughly in cold water until the water runs clear.
2. Cook the rice in a rice cooker or on the stovetop with 2 cups of water and a pinch of salt. Once cooked, spread the rice on a plate to cool.

Ingredients for Karuveppilai (Curry Leaf) Paste:

- 1 cup fresh curry leaves, washed and pat-dried
- 2-3 red chilies (adjust to your spice preference)
- 1/4 cup grated coconut (fresh or frozen)
- 1/2 teaspoon cumin seeds (jeera)
- A small piece of ginger (about 1/2 inch)
- 1-2 tablespoons water (for grinding)
- Salt to taste

Instructions:

For Karuveppilai (Curry Leaf) Paste:

1. In a blender or food processor, combine fresh curry leaves, red chilies, grated coconut, cumin seeds, ginger, and a pinch of salt.
2. Add 1-2 tablespoons of water to the blender and grind everything into a smooth paste. The paste should have a thick but spreadable consistency.

You need for Seasoning:

- 2 tablespoons ghee (clarified butter) or coconut oil (for a vegan option)
- 1/2 teaspoon mustard seeds
- 1/2 teaspoon urad dal (split black gram)
- A pinch of asafoetida (hing)
- A few cashew nuts (optional, for garnish)
- Fresh curry leaves for garnish (optional)

Instructions:

For Karuveppilai (Curry Leaf) Paste:

3. In a blender or food processor, combine fresh curry leaves, red chilies, grated coconut, cumin seeds, ginger, and a pinch of salt.
4. Add 1-2 tablespoons of water to the blender and grind everything into a smooth paste. The paste should have a thick but spreadable consistency.

Instructions for seasoning and assembly:

1. Heat ghee or coconut oil in a pan over medium heat.
2. Add mustard seeds and let them splutter.
3. Add urad dal and sauté until it turns golden brown.
4. Add a pinch of asafoetida and cashew nuts (if using). Sauté for a minute until the cashews turn tan brown.
5. Reduce the heat to low and add the curry leaf paste. Stir well and cook for 2-3 minutes. The paste should release its aroma.
6. Add the cooked rice to the pan and gently mix it with the paste until the rice is well coated. You can use a fork to separate the rice grains if needed.
7. Adjust salt to taste and continue to cook for another 2-3 minutes to heat the rice through.
8. Garnish the Karuveppilai Rice with fresh curry leaves (if using).
9. Remove from heat and serve hot.

Serving Suggestion

Medhoo Vada https://youtu.be/BQSYBuqWi2o

Brussels Sprout Quiche https://youtu.be/7BXgc3C7X4w

Asparagus fry https://youtu.be/iFhUXipK-t8

12. Mangalore Buns

Mangalore Buns, also known simply as "Buns," are a popular breakfast or tea-time snack from the coastal region of Mangalore in Karnataka, India. They are sweet, fluffy, and slightly crispy on the outside. Banana meets bun in this oh-so-sweet south Indian snack. Mashed up banana with dough, curd, sugar, salt, cumin seeds and baking soda, is set aside for a few hours. Then, it's heated up with some oil in a pan, made into little round pooris and ultimately dunked into the hot oil all the best street food seems to emerge from. Mangalore Buns are a delightful treat with a unique sweet and slightly savory flavor.

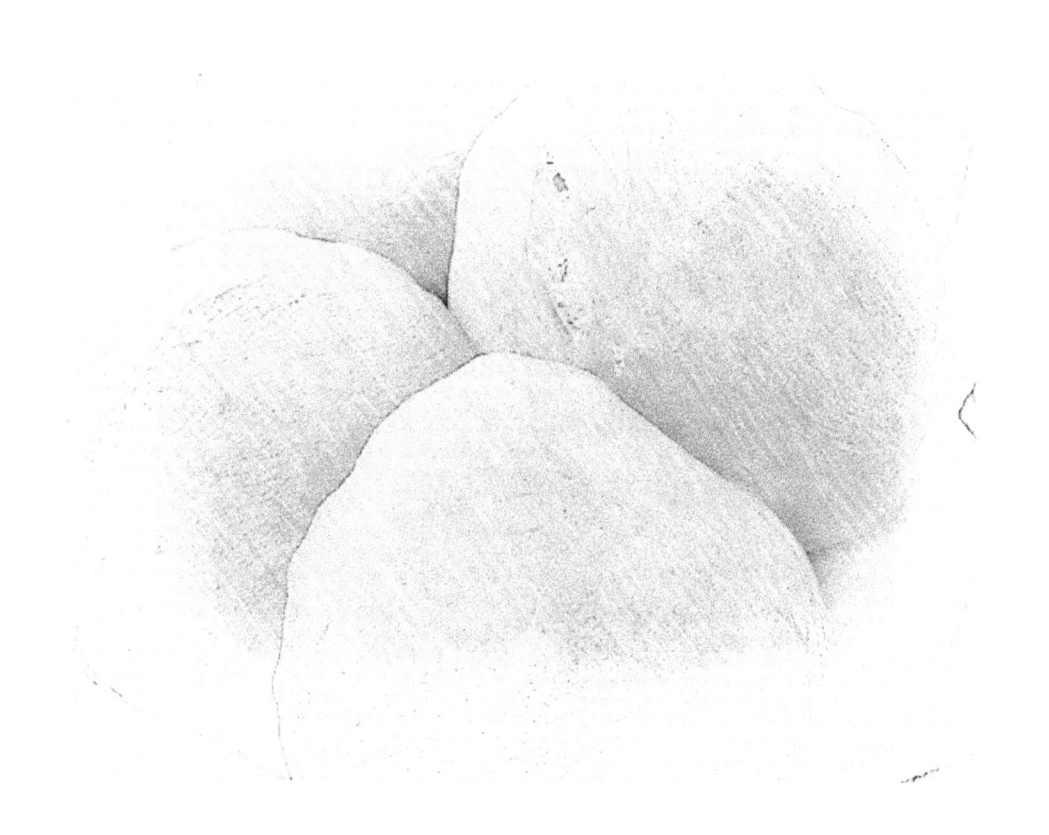

Ingredients:

For the Dough:

- 2 ripe bananas (medium-sized)
- 2 cups all-purpose flour (maida)
- 1/4 cup yogurt (curd)
- 2 tablespoons sugar
- 1/2 teaspoon salt
- 1/2 teaspoon baking soda
- A pinch of turmeric powder (for color)
- A pinch of cardamom powder (optional, for flavor)
- Oil for deep frying
- Water (as needed)

Instructions:

1. Peel the ripe bananas and mash them well in a mixing bowl until there are no lumps.
2. To the mashed bananas, add sugar, salt, baking soda, turmeric powder, and cardamom powder (if using). Mix everything together.
3. Gradually add the all-purpose flour to the banana mixture and mix it well.
4. Add yogurt to the mixture and continue to knead until a soft and pliable dough forms. If the dough is too dry, you can add a little water to make it soft. The dough should be slightly sticky but not too wet.
5. Cover the dough with a damp cloth or plastic wrap and let it rest for about 2-3 hours. This resting time allows the dough to ferment slightly and become airy.
6. After the resting period, divide the dough into small lemon-sized portions.

7. Roll each portion into a ball and flatten it slightly to form a bun or small disc. You can use a rolling pin to flatten them, but they should be thicker than regular chapatis.
8. Heat oil in a deep frying pan or kadai over medium heat. The oil should be hot but not smoking.
9. Carefully slide the shaped buns into the hot oil, one or two at a time, depending on the size of your pan.
10. Fry the buns until they turn golden brown and puff up, turning them occasionally for even cooking. This should take about 3-4 minutes per batch.
11. Remove the fried Mangalore Buns from the oil using a slotted spoon and place them on paper towels to drain excess oil.
12. Serve the Mangalore Buns hot. They are best enjoyed fresh and crispy.

Serving Suggestions:

Ginger cucumber relish https://youtu.be/cvPbFuWJV8E

Sattvic Puzhukku https://youtu.be/E5Di-leC46s

Sattvic Brinjal Sambar https://youtu.be/wyqNKz74tzU

13. Mango Rice

Mango Rice, also known as "Maanga Sadam" in South India, is a delicious and tangy rice dish made with ripe mangoes, rice, and a blend of spices. It's a flavorful and popular South Indian recipe, especially during the mango season. Mango Rice is a delightful blend of sweet, tangy, and spicy flavors. It's perfect for lunch or as a side dish at any time of the day, especially during the mango season. Enjoy!

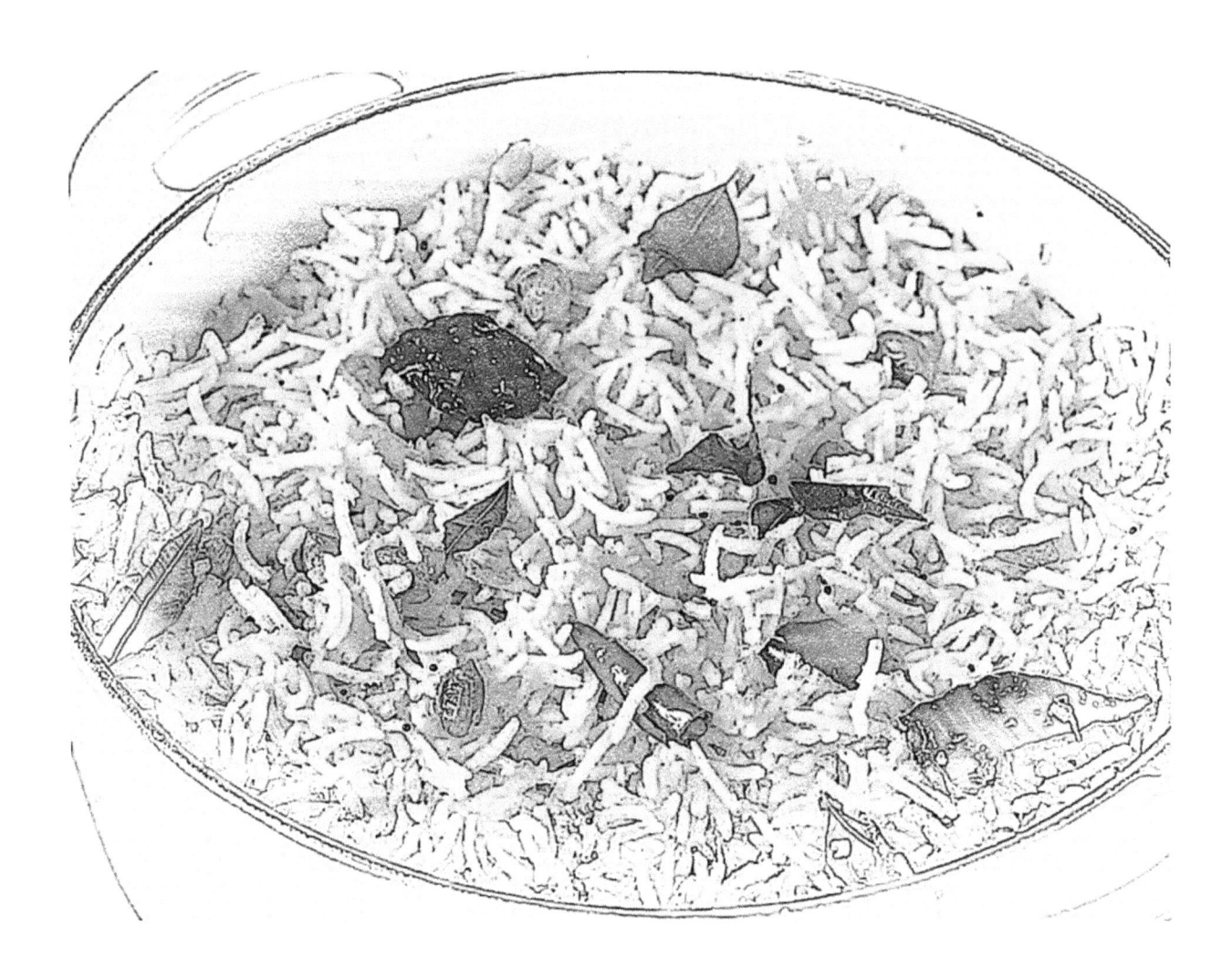

Ingredients:

- 1 cup basmati rice or any long-grain rice
- 2 ripe mangoes
- 2-3 tablespoons oil
- 1/2 teaspoon mustard seeds
- 1/2 teaspoon urad dal (split black gram)
- 1/2 teaspoon chana dal (split chickpeas)
- A pinch of asafoetida (hing)
- 2-3 red chilies, chopped (adjust to your spice preference)
- 10-12 curry leaves
- 1/4 teaspoon turmeric powder
- Salt to taste
- 2-3 tablespoons grated coconut (fresh or frozen)
- A few cashew nuts (optional, for garnish)
- Fresh coriander leaves for garnish (optional)

Instructions:

1. Wash the rice thoroughly and cook it with the appropriate amount of water until it's fluffy and each grain is separate. You can use a rice cooker or cook it on the stovetop. Once it's cooked, spread it on a plate to cool.

2. Wash and peel the ripe mangoes. Remove the flesh from the seeds and chop it into small pieces. You can also mash some of the mango pieces to add more mango flavor.

3. Take about half of the chopped mango pieces and blend them into a smooth paste using a blender or food processor. Set this mango paste aside.

4. Heat oil in a large pan or kadai over medium heat. Add mustard seeds and let them splutter.

5. Add urad dal and chana dal. Sauté until they turn golden brown. Add a pinch of asafoetida, chopped red chilies, and curry leaves. Sauté for a minute until the chilies become slightly soft. Add turmeric powder and sauté for a few seconds.

6. Now, add the mango paste to the pan and cook it for 2-3 minutes until it thickens and the raw mango aroma diminishes. Add salt to taste and mix well.

7. Add the cooked rice to the mango mixture and gently mix it until the rice is well coated with the mango paste.

8. Finally, add the remaining chopped mango pieces, grated coconut, and fresh coriander leaves. Mix everything together.

9. If you want, you can roast some cashew nuts in a little ghee and garnish the Mango Rice with them. Remove the Mango Rice from the heat and let it cool slightly. Serve the Mango Rice warm or at room temperature.

Serving Suggestions

Apple thokku https://youtu.be/kLpvFTfA4Qk

Easy eggplant https://youtu.be/AGL5wHML_iM

Cabbage quiche https://youtu.be/chzU5CdRdlo

14. Masala Dosa

Masala Dosa is a popular South Indian dish consisting of a crispy fermented rice and urad dal (black gram) crepe filled with a spiced potato filling. It's often served with coconut chutney and sambar.

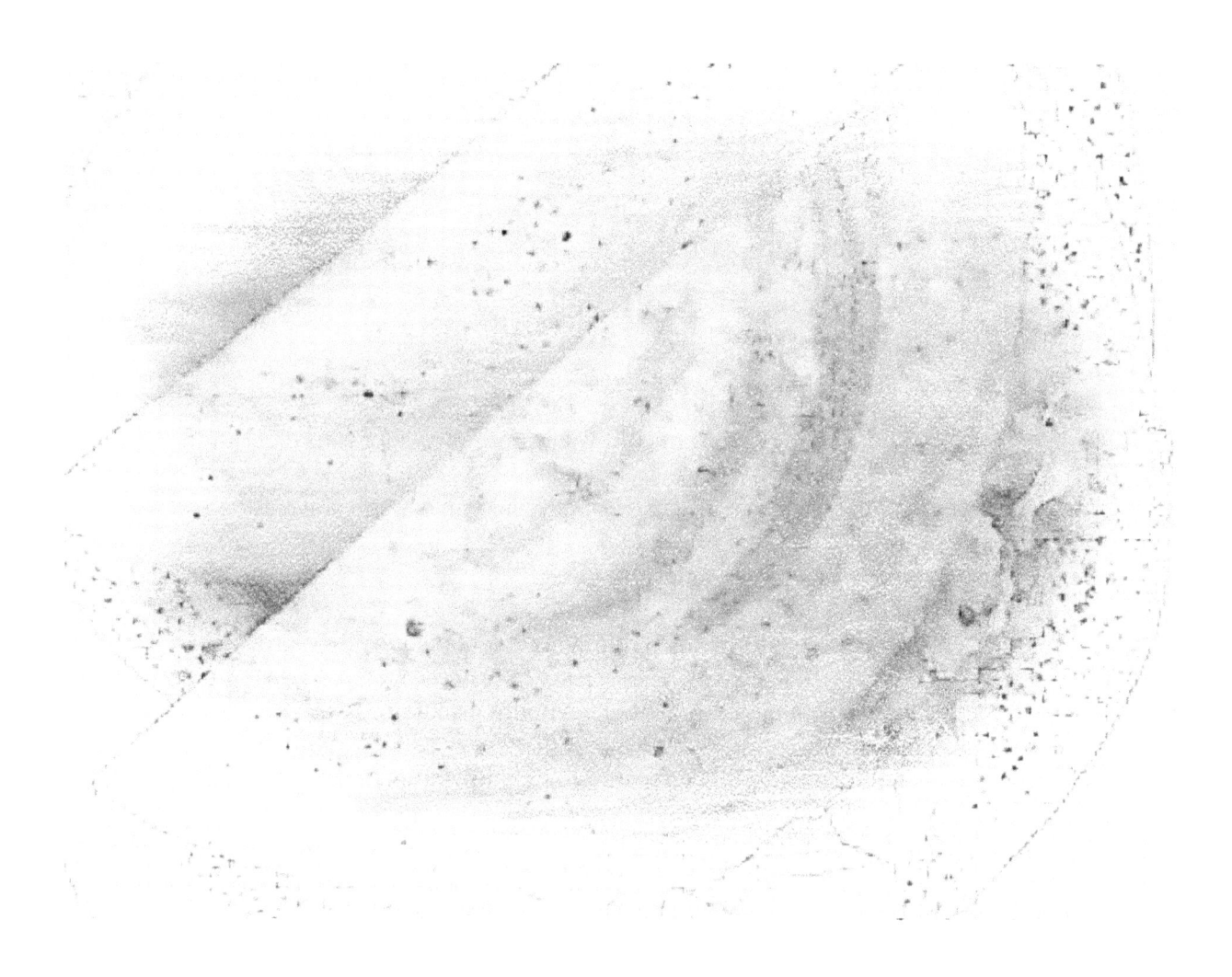

Ingredients:

For the Dosa Batter:

- 1 cup long-grain parboiled rice (Idli rice) or regular rice
- 1/4 cup urad dal (split black gram)
- 1/4 teaspoon fenugreek seeds (methi seeds)
- Salt to taste
- Water (for grinding)

Instructions:

To make the Dosa Batter:

1. Wash the rice and urad dal together in cold water until the water runs clear. Add fenugreek seeds to the washed rice and dal. Soak them in enough water for about 4-6 hours or overnight.
2. Drain the soaked rice and dal mixture. Add them to a blender or food processor.
3. Add enough water to the blender to facilitate smooth grinding. Grind the rice and dal mixture into a smooth batter. The batter should be thick but pourable. Add salt and mix well.
4. Transfer the batter to a large bowl and let it ferment in a warm place for 8-12 hours or until it's doubled in volume. The fermentation time may vary depending on the temperature of your surroundings.

For the Potato Filling:

- 3-4 medium-sized potatoes, boiled, peeled, and mashed
- 1 cup peas
- 2-3 red chilies, finely chopped (adjust to your spice preference)
- 1/2 teaspoon mustard seeds
- 1/2 teaspoon cumin seeds (jeera)
- A pinch of asafoetida (hing)
- A few curry leaves
- 1/2 teaspoon turmeric powder
- Salt to taste
- 2 tablespoons oil
- Fresh coriander leaves, chopped (for garnish)

Instructions:

For Potato Filling:

1. Heat oil in a pan over medium heat. Add mustard seeds, red chilies, cumin seeds, and a pinch of asafoetida. Let the seeds splutter.
2. Add curry leaves and turmeric powder. Mix well.
3. Add the peas, mashed potatoes, and salt. Mix everything together until well combined.
4. Cook for a few minutes until the potato filling is heated through and flavors are well blended. Remove from heat.

To make Masala Dosa:

1. Heat a non-stick dosa tava (griddle) or a flat pan over medium heat. Grease it lightly with oil.

2. Pour a ladleful of the dosa batter onto the center of the hot tava.
3. Quickly spread the batter in a circular motion to form a thin dosa. The dosa should be thin and crispy.
4. Drizzle a little oil over the dosa and around the edges.
5. When the dosa turns golden brown and crispy on the bottom, spread a portion of the prepared potato filling over one half of the dosa.
6. Gently fold the other half over the filling, creating a semi-circular shape.
7. Cook for a minute or two until the dosa is crisp and golden brown on both sides.
8. Remove the Masala Dosa from the tava and serve hot.

Serving Suggestions:

Tomato gojju https://youtu.be/o3puB6btxaE

Ghee https://youtu.be/s6hL61F5BSQ

Apple thokku https://youtu.be/kLpvFTfA4Qk

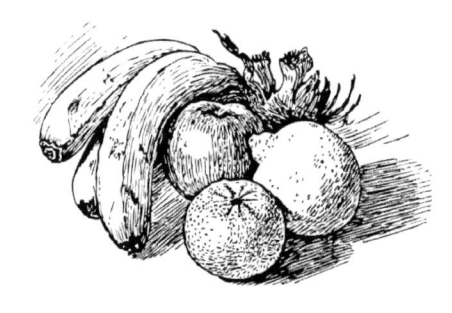

15. Moong Dal Dosa

Moong Dal Dosa is a nutritious and protein-rich variation of the traditional dosa. It's made using moong dal (split red gram) instead of the usual rice and urad dal batter. Moong Dal Dosa is a healthy and tasty alternative to traditional dosas. It's especially great for those looking to incorporate more protein into their diet.

Ingredients:

You need for Batter:

- 1 cup split moong dal (red gram)
- 1/4 cup rice flour (optional, for crispiness)
- 2-3 red chilies (adjust to your spice preference)
- A small piece of ginger
- A handful of fresh coriander leaves
- 1/2 teaspoon cumin seeds (jeera)
- A pinch of asafoetida (hing)
- Salt to taste
- Water (as needed for grinding)

Instructions:

To Prepare the Batter:

1. Wash the split moong dal thoroughly under running water. Soak it in enough water for about 4-5 hours.
2. Drain the soaked moong dal and add it to a blender or food processor.
3. Add red chilies, ginger, fresh coriander leaves, cumin seeds, asafoetida, and salt to the dal.
4. Blend everything together, gradually adding water as needed to make a smooth batter. The consistency should be similar to regular dosa batter.
5. If you want your dosas to be crisper, you can add rice flour to the batter and mix it in thoroughly.

To make Moong Dal Dosa:

1. Heat a non-stick dosa tava or a regular frying pan over medium heat. You can lightly grease it with oil or use it as is.
2. Once the tava is hot, pour a ladleful of the moong dal batter onto the center of the tava.
3. Quickly spread the batter in a circular motion to form a thin dosa. It doesn't need to be as thin as a traditional dosa, but it should be spread evenly.
4. Sprinkle your choice of seasoning on top, such as finely chopped green onions, fresh coriander leaves, grated coconut, and chopped red chilies.
5. Drizzle a few drops of oil around the edges of the dosa and a little on top.
6. Cook the dosa on medium heat until it turns golden brown and crispy on the bottom.
7. Flip the dosa and cook the other side until it's golden brown as well.
8. Remove the moong dal dosa from the tava and serve it hot.
9. Repeat the process for the remaining batter, adjusting the seasoning as desired.

Serving suggestions;

Apple chutney https://youtu.be/1vKLKDKxym0

Potato saagu https://youtu.be/jlQ8FMdr7dA

Raita https://youtu.be/Svd7w-MsLd8

16. Neer Dosa

Neer Dosa is a popular South Indian crepe made from a thin rice batter. It's known for its soft and delicate texture and is typically served with coconut chutney or a variety of other side dishes.

You need:

- 1 cup rice (preferably sona masuri or any medium-grain rice)
- 1/4 cup grated coconut (fresh or frozen)
- Salt to taste
- Water for grinding (approximately 1.5 to 2 cups)

Instructions:

1. Wash the rice thoroughly in cold water until the water runs clear.
2. Soak the washed rice in enough water for about 4-6 hours or overnight.
3. Drain the soaked rice and place it in a blender or food processor.
4. Add the grated coconut and a pinch of salt to the rice.
5. Start by adding about 1.5 cups of water to the blender. You can adjust the water quantity as needed to achieve a thin and runny batter.
6. Blend everything together until you get a smooth batter. The consistency should be thinner than regular dosa batter and almost watery.
7. Transfer the batter to a large bowl and let it rest for about 30 minutes. This allows the rice to settle at the bottom, and you can pour the thinner batter on top.
8. Heat a non-stick or well-seasoned crepe pan over medium heat. You don't need to add oil to the pan.
9. Stir the batter gently to ensure it's well mixed.
10. Ladle a small amount of batter into the center of the hot pan (about 1/4 cup or less, depending on the size of your pan).

11. Quickly swirl the pan to spread the batter into a thin, circular shape. Neer Dosa should be thin and have small holes.

12. Cover the pan with a lid and let the dosa cook for about 1-2 minutes. It cooks quickly due to its thinness. There's no need to flip the dosa as it cooks only on one side.

13. When the edges start to lift off the pan and the center looks cooked, remove the dosa from the pan and place it on a plate.

14. Serve the Neer Dosa hot with coconut chutney, tomato chutney, or any chutney of your choice. You can also serve it with a side of vegetable curry.

Serving suggestions

Sampangi Pitlay https://youtu.be/n9qZ_EhkM-Q

Sambar https://youtu.be/wyqNKz74tzU

Parsley chutney https://youtu.be/ADth8ETWRR8

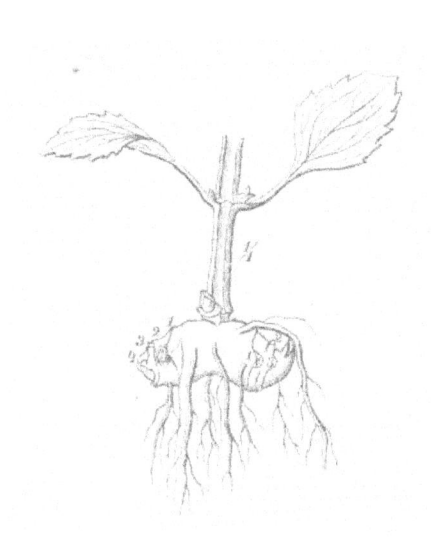

17. Pazhampori

Pazhampori, also known as Ethakka Appam, is a popular South Indian snack made from ripe bananas, preferably Kerala bananas, also known as Nendran or Ethakka. These bananas are sliced, coated in a sweet and spiced batter, and deep-fried until they are golden and crispy. Pazhampori is a delightful treat with a sweet and slightly spicy flavor. The crispiness of the fried batter complements the sweetness of the ripe bananas perfectly. Enjoy your homemade Pazhampori!

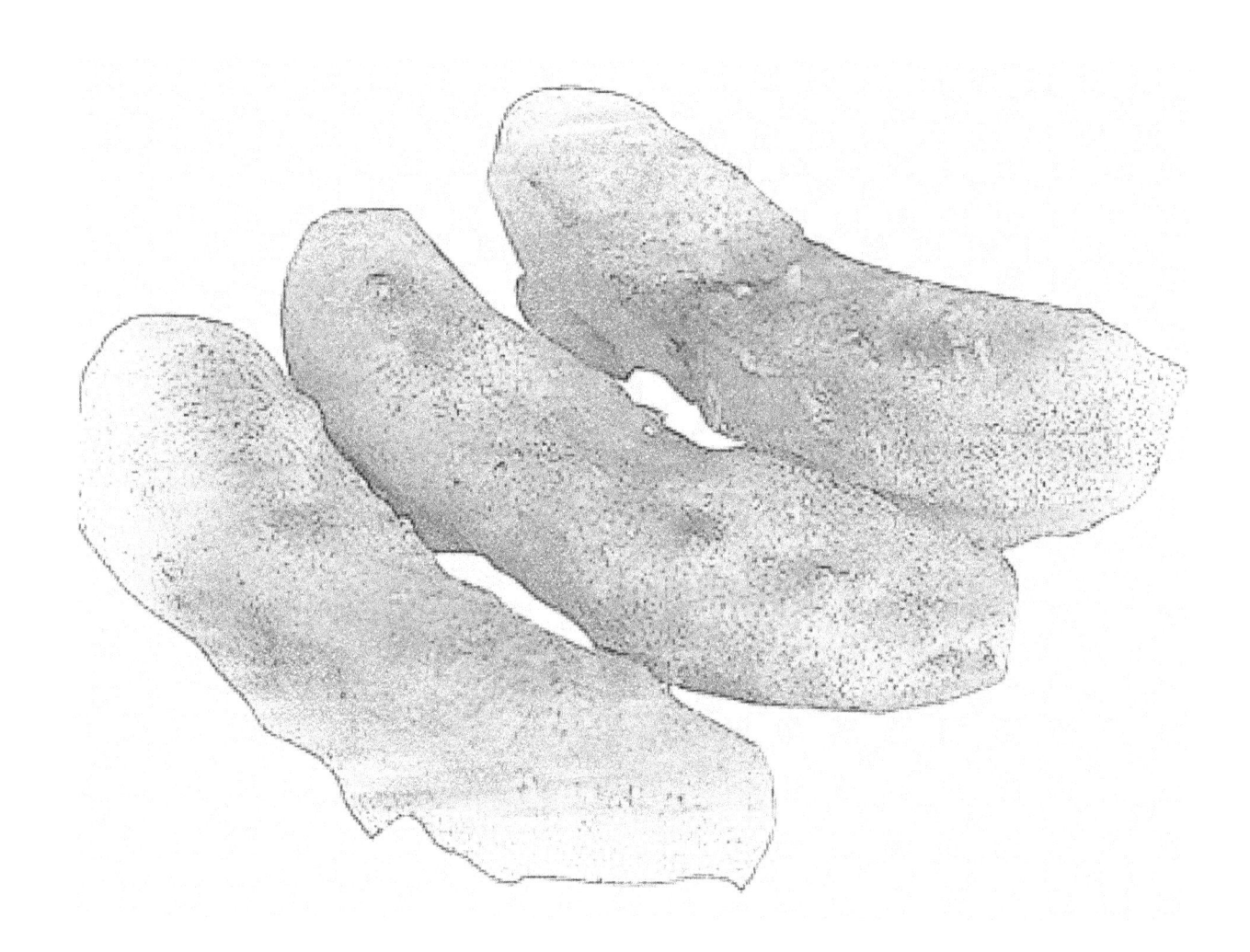

Ingredients:

- 2 ripe bananas
- 1 cup all-purpose flour (maida)
- 2 tablespoons rice flour
- 2 tablespoons sugar (optional
- 1/4 teaspoon turmeric powder
- ¼ teaspoon cardamom powder
- A pinch of salt
- Water (as needed to make a thick batter)
- Oil for deep frying

Instructions:

1. In a mixing bowl, combine the all-purpose flour, rice flour, sugar, turmeric powder (if using), cardamom powder, and a pinch of salt. Mix everything together.
2. Gradually add water while stirring to make a thick batter. The batter should be thick enough to coat the back of a spoon. It should not be too thin.
3. Peel the ripe bananas and cut them into thin, elongated slices. Ensure that the slices are not too thick; they should be thin enough to cook through when fried.
4. Dip each banana slice into the batter, ensuring that it's well-coated on all sides.
5. Heat oil in a deep frying pan or kadai over medium heat. To check if the oil is hot enough, drop a small amount of batter into the oil. If it sizzles and rises to the top, the oil is ready for frying.
6. Carefully slide the coated banana slices into the hot oil. Fry them in batches to avoid overcrowding the pan.
7. Fry the banana slices until they turn golden brown and crispy on both sides. Use a slotted spoon to flip them occasionally for even cooking.

8. Once they are golden brown and crispy, remove the Pazhampuri from the oil and drain them on a paper towel to remove excess oil.

9. Serve the Pazhampuri hot as a side dish. They are often enjoyed with a cup of tea or coffee.

Serving suggestions:

Pazhampori is usually eaten with chai (tea) or coffee, usually on the go. You can make it a part of a hearty breakfast by pairing with the following items-

Chai https://youtu.be/ywzwbVgxkeM

Milk Peda https://youtu.be/TOeAz0sHh-E

Millet-Mango Kanji https://youtu.be/Et70Yy9ks_o

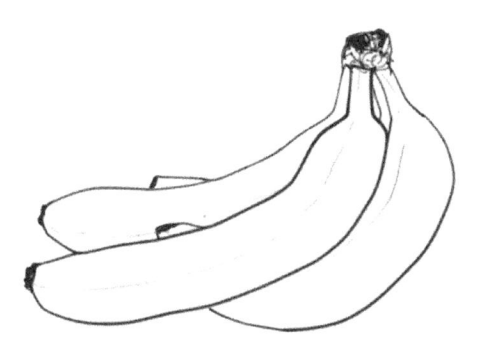

18. Paniyaram

Paniyaram is a popular South Indian snack made from fermented rice and lentil batter. They are typically cooked in a special pan with depressions or molds, which gives them their unique round shape.

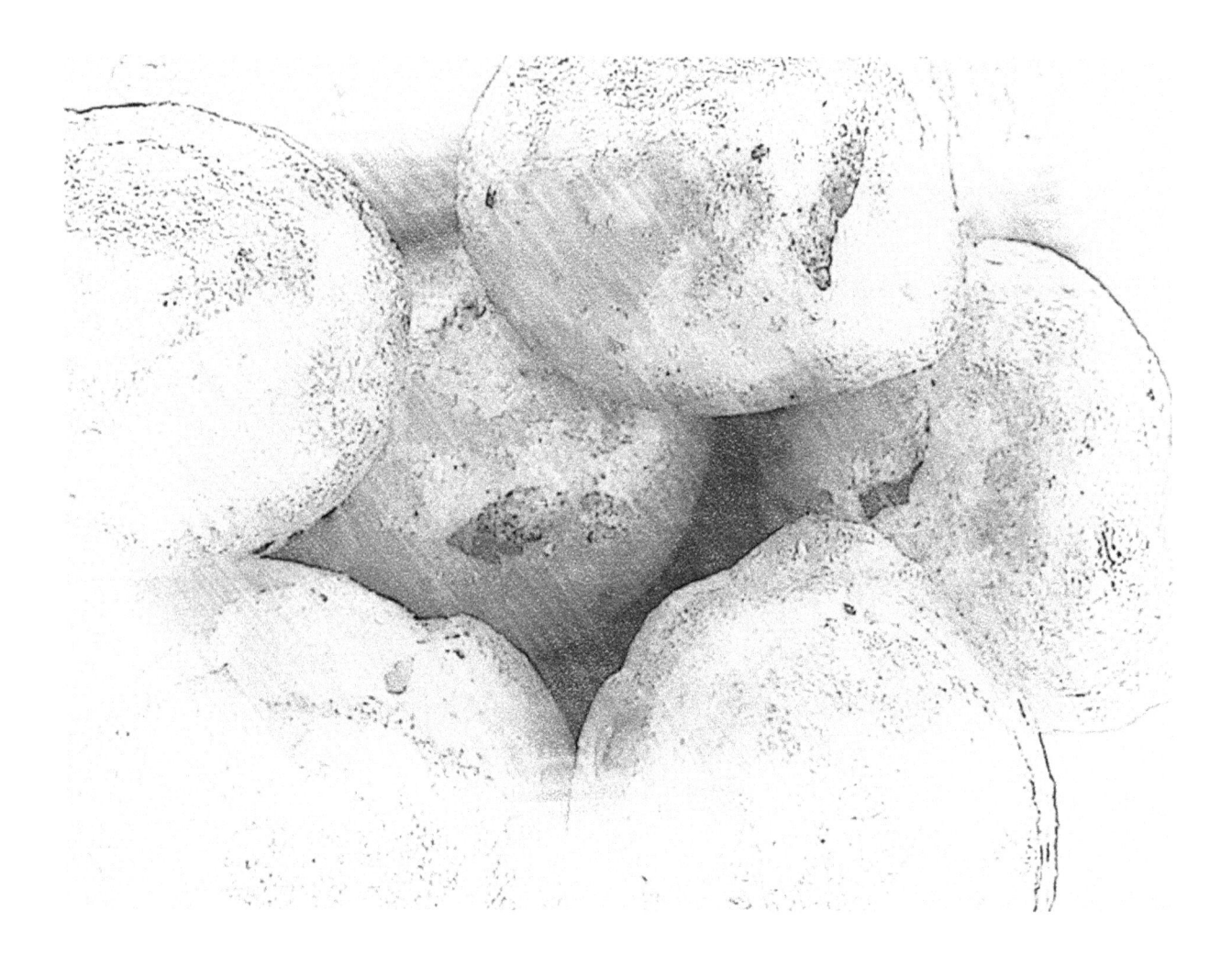

Ingredients:

For the Batter:

- 1 cup idli rice or regular rice
- 1/4 cup urad dal (split black gram)
- 1/4 cup chana dal (split chickpeas)
- 1/2 teaspoon methi seeds
- A pinch of asafoetida (hing)
- Salt to taste
- Water for grinding

Instructions:

To Prepare the Batter:

1. Wash the rice, urad dal, chana dal, and fenugreek seeds together under running water until the water runs clear. Soak them in enough water for about 4-6 hours.
2. Drain the soaked rice and dals. Then, grind them into a smooth batter using as little water as possible. The batter should be thick and have a texture similar to that of dosa batter.
3. Add a pinch of asafoetida and salt to the batter. Mix well.
4. Cover the batter and let it ferment overnight or for at least 6-8 hours. The fermentation time may vary depending on the temperature of your surroundings. The batter should rise and become slightly frothy when it's ready.

For Seasoning:

- 1 large carrot, finely chopped
- 2-3 red chilies, finely chopped (adjust to your spice preference)
- A few curry leaves, chopped
- A small piece of ginger, grated
- 2 tablespoons chopped fresh cilantro leaves
- Oil for cooking

Instructions:

To make Paniyaram:

1. Heat a Paniyaram pan (also known as an appe pan or aebleskiver pan) over medium heat. Add a few drops of oil in each cup.
2. While the pan is heating, add the finely chopped cilantro, red chilies, grated carrot, grated ginger, chopped curry leaves to the fermented batter. Mix everything together.
3. Once the pan is hot, pour a spoonful of the batter into each depression. Fill them to about 3/4 full, as the Paniyarams will puff up while cooking.
4. Cover the pan with a lid and cook the Paniyarams on medium heat for about 2-3 minutes.
5. When the sides turn golden brown and crispy, flip the Paniyarams using a skewer or a spoon.
6. Cook the other side for an additional 2-3 minutes, or until they become golden brown and cooked through.
7. Remove the Paniyarams from the pan and place them on a plate.

Serving suggestions:

Ghee https://youtu.be/s6hL61F5BSQ

Apple thokku https://youtu.be/kLpvFTfA4Qk

Gojju https://youtu.be/o3puB6btxaE

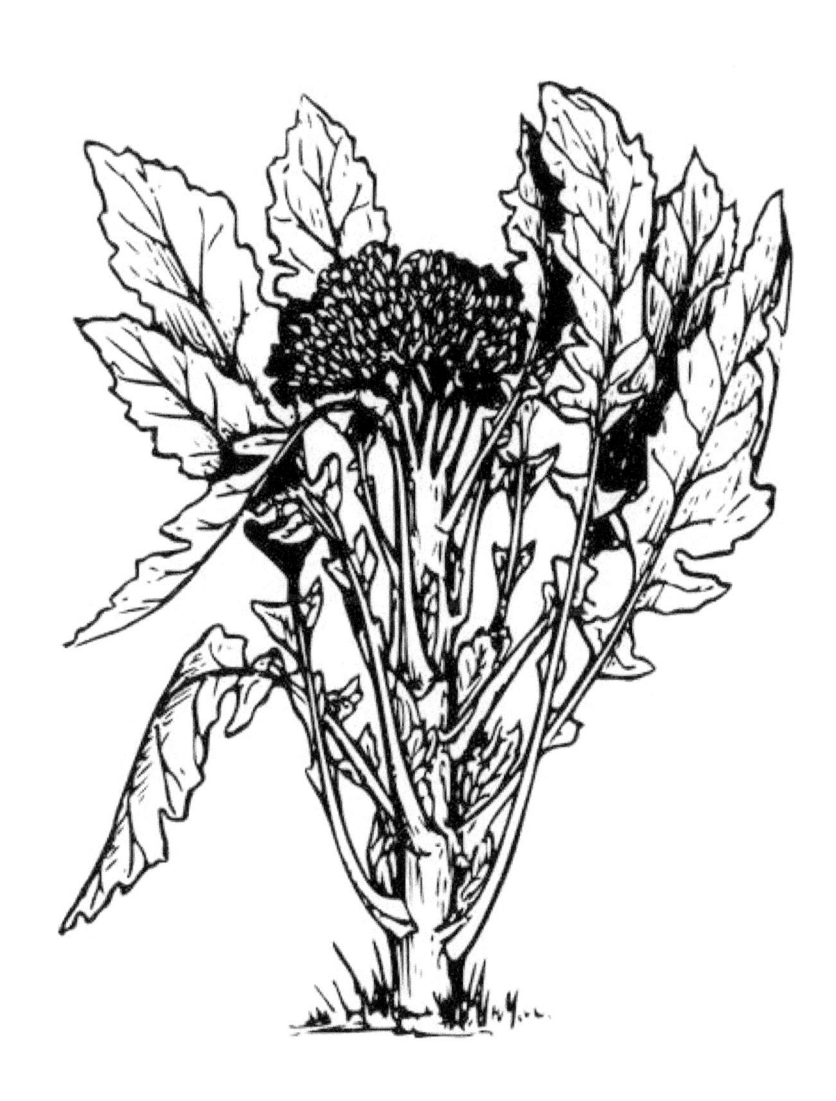

19. Punugulu- Minapappu

Minapappu Punugulu, also known as Urad Dal Fritters, is a popular South Indian snack that's crispy and crunchy on the outside and soft on the inside. They are made from urad dal (black gram) and rice, and they are deliciously spiced.

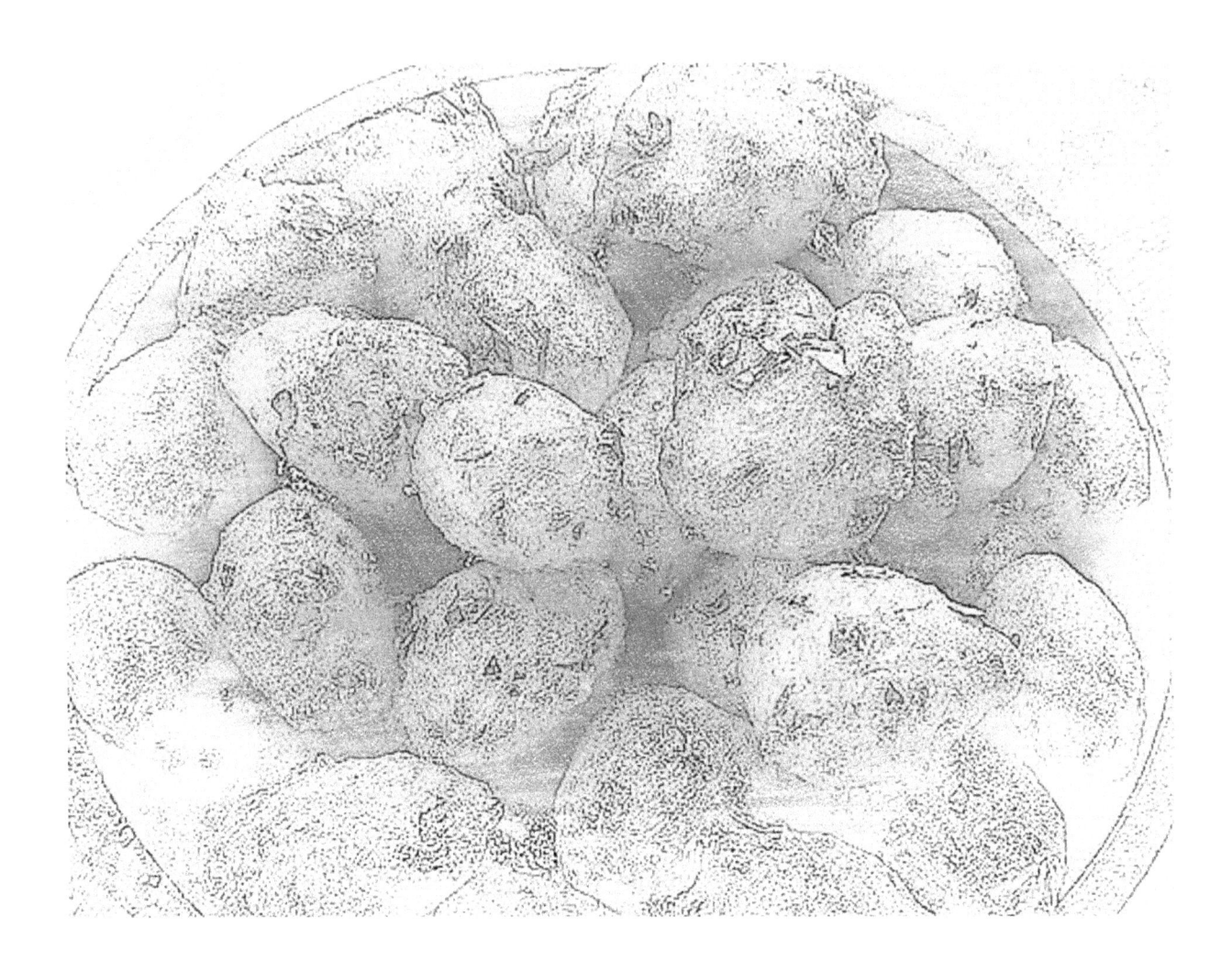

Ingredients:

For Batter:

- 1 cup urad dal (black gram)
- 1/4 cup rice
- 1-2 red chilies (adjust to your spice preference)
- 1-inch piece of ginger
- A pinch of asafoetida (hing)
- Salt to taste
- Water, as needed

For Tempering:

- 1 medium-sized green onion bunch, finely chopped
- 1-2 red chilies, finely cut
- A few curry leaves, finely chopped
- 2 tablespoons fresh coriander leaves, chopped (optional)
- Oil for deep frying

Instructions:

1. Wash the urad dal and rice thoroughly, and then soak them together in enough water for about 3-4 hours. This helps in easy grinding.

2. Drain the soaked urad dal and rice. Grind them together with red chilies, ginger, asafoetida, and a little water to a smooth and thick batter. The batter should be of a dropping consistency, not too runny. Add salt and mix well.

3. In a separate pan, heat a tablespoon of oil. Add finely chopped red onions, red chilies, and curry leaves. Sauté and add chopped cilantro leaves for extra flavor.

4. Add the sautéed mixture to the urad dal batter and mix well. This step adds a delicious crunch and flavor to the Punugulu.

5. Heat oil in a deep frying pan over medium heat. To check if the oil is hot enough, drop a small amount of batter into the oil. If it sizzles and rises to the surface, the oil is ready.

6. Wet your hands with a little water to prevent the batter from sticking. Take small portions of the batter and shape them into lemon-sized round or oval fritters. You can make these fritters as big or small as you like.

7. Fry the fritters in batches. Carefully slide them into the hot oil and fry until they turn golden brown and crispy on the outside. It usually takes about 3-4 minutes per batch.

8. Make sure not to overcrowd the pan, as it can reduce the oil temperature and make the fritters absorb more oil.

9. Once they are golden brown and crisp, use a slotted spoon to remove them from the oil. Place them on a plate lined with paper towels to remove excess oil.

Serving suggestions:

Idli https://www.youtube.com/watch?v=kxPtx8Z4-Tw

Dosa https://youtu.be/hmueE_40RdU

Upma https://youtu.be/UeMTRcyz6MA

20. Puttu

Puttu is a traditional South Indian breakfast dish made from steamed rice flour and grated coconut. It is made in a special vessel puttu steamer or a steaming vessel with a perforated. You can also make it in small cups. It's typically served with kadala curry (black chickpea curry), but it can also be enjoyed with other curries or even with sugar and ripe bananas.

To enjoy Puttu, you can crumble it on your plate, add a spoonful of kadala curry or your preferred curry, and mix it well before eating. It's a simple yet delicious South Indian breakfast dish that's a favorite among many.

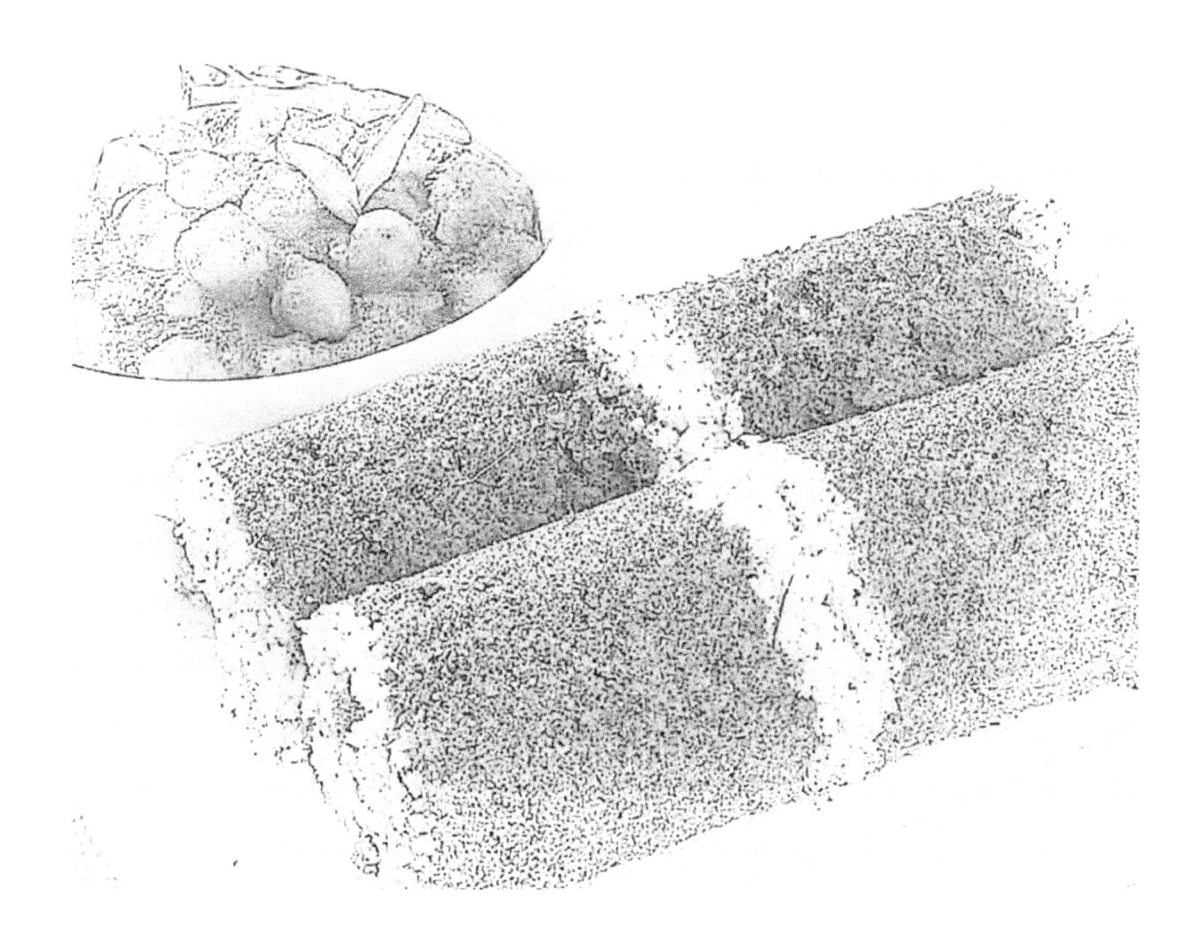

Ingredients:

For Making Puttu:

- 1 cup rice flour
- 1/4 cup grated coconut (fresh or frozen)
- Water (approximately 1/2 to 3/4 cup, as needed)
- A pinch of salt

Instructions:

Preparing the Puttu Mixture:

1. Take the rice flour in a mixing bowl. Add a pinch of salt and mix well.
2. Gradually add water while mixing with your fingers. Keep adding water in small quantities until the rice flour becomes damp and crumbly. It should not be too wet; just enough to hold its shape when pressed together.
3. Break up any lumps in the mixture with your fingers. The texture should resemble bread crumbs.

Layering the Puttu:

1. If you have a Puttu maker, place the perforated plate at the bottom of the cylindrical portion.
2. Start by adding a layer of grated coconut to the bottom of the cylindrical portion. This is optional but adds a nice coconut flavor to the Puttu.

3. Next, add a layer of the prepared rice flour mixture. Alternate layers of rice flour mixture and grated coconut until the cylinder is filled, ending with a layer of rice flour on top.
4. Cover the top of the cylindrical portion with a thin, clean cloth or a piece of muslin cloth.

Steaming the Puttu:

1. Place the cylindrical portion onto the steaming vessel with water in it. Make sure it fits snugly.
2. Steam the Puttu on medium heat for about 10-12 minutes or until it's cooked. You will see steam escaping from the top holes of the Puttu maker when it's done.
3. Remove the Puttu maker from the steaming vessel and carefully push the cooked Puttu onto a plate using a wooden stick or a long spoon.
4. Serve the Puttu hot with kadala curry, sugar, or any curry of your choice.

Serving suggestions for Puttu:

Cholae https://youtu.be/t4j5wIurDV8

Chakka Varatti https://youtu.be/uy7KIRvm7v0

Carrot Chutney https://youtu.be/gtBSNX51YPg

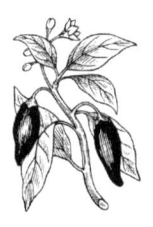

21. Rava Kesari

Rava Kesari is a popular South Indian dessert made from semolina (rava or sooji), sugar, ghee, and flavored with cardamom and saffron. It's known for its beautiful orange color and delicious taste. Rava Kesari is a delightful Indian dessert that's loved by people of all ages. It's often served during festivals and special occasions. Enjoy it warm or at room temperature.

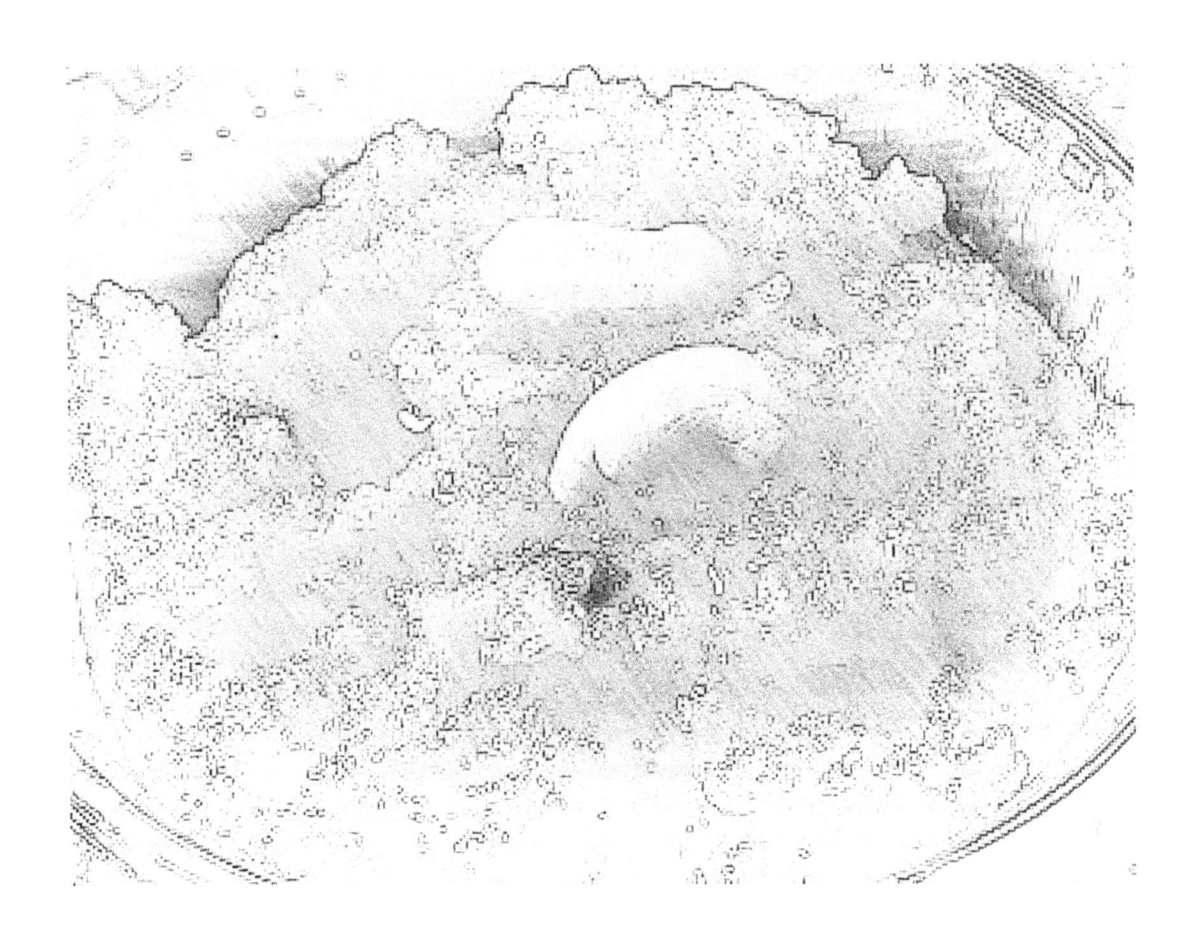

Ingredients:

- 1 cup fine semolina (rava or sooji)
- 1 cup sugar
- 1/4 cup ghee (clarified butter)
- 1/4 cup chopped cashew nuts
- A pinch of saffron strands (optional)
- 1/2 teaspoon cardamom powder
- A few raisins (optional)
- A few drops of orange food color (optional)
- 2 1/2 cups water
- A pinch of salt

Instructions:

1. **To prepare Saffron Infusion (Optional):** If you're using saffron strands, soak them in 2 tablespoons of warm milk and set them aside for about 10-15 minutes to release their color and flavor.
2. Heat a heavy-bottomed pan or kadai over low-medium heat and add the semolina. Dry roast it while continuously stirring for about 5-7 minutes until it turns aromatic and slightly changes color. Be careful not to brown it too much; it should remain pale.
3. In a separate saucepan, heat 2 ½ cups of water. Bring it to a boil, then reduce the heat to low and keep it simmering.
4. In the same pan used for roasting semolina, add the ghee and chopped cashew nuts. Sauté the cashews until they turn golden brown. You can also add raisins at this stage if you like.
5. Once the cashews are roasted, add the roasted semolina to the pan. Mix well to combine the ghee and semolina.

6. Gradually add the sugar to the semolina mixture and keep stirring. The sugar will melt and the mixture will become watery. Use as little sugar as possible as sugar is not considered sattvic

7. If you soaked saffron strands, add them along with the saffron-infused milk to the mixture. Add cardamom powder for flavor. Also, add a pinch of salt to balance the sweetness.

8. Continue stirring the mixture over low-medium heat. The semolina will absorb the water and thicken.

9. If you want to give your Rava Kesari a vibrant orange color, add a few drops of orange food color at this stage. This is optional and can be omitted.

10. Keep stirring and cooking the mixture until it leaves the sides of the pan and forms a thick mass. It should take about 5-7 minutes.

11. Once the Rava Kesari is ready, remove it from the heat and transfer it to a greased plate or dish. Flatten it with a spatula and allow it to cool for a few minutes.

12. Once it has cooled slightly, cut the Rava Kesari into pieces or squares and serve.

Serving Suggestions:

Aama vadai https://youtu.be/sJ3tfA1dJ4Q

Cabbage pakoda https://youtu.be/vY4jSb13fGI

Bonda https://youtu.be/N5NvBE-RSgI

22. Rava idli

Rava Idli is a popular South Indian dish made from semolina (rava) and yogurt, often served as a quick and easy breakfast option. It doesn't require fermentation like traditional rice-based idlis. Rava Idlis are soft, fluffy, and have a delightful texture. Enjoy them as a breakfast option or as a snack.

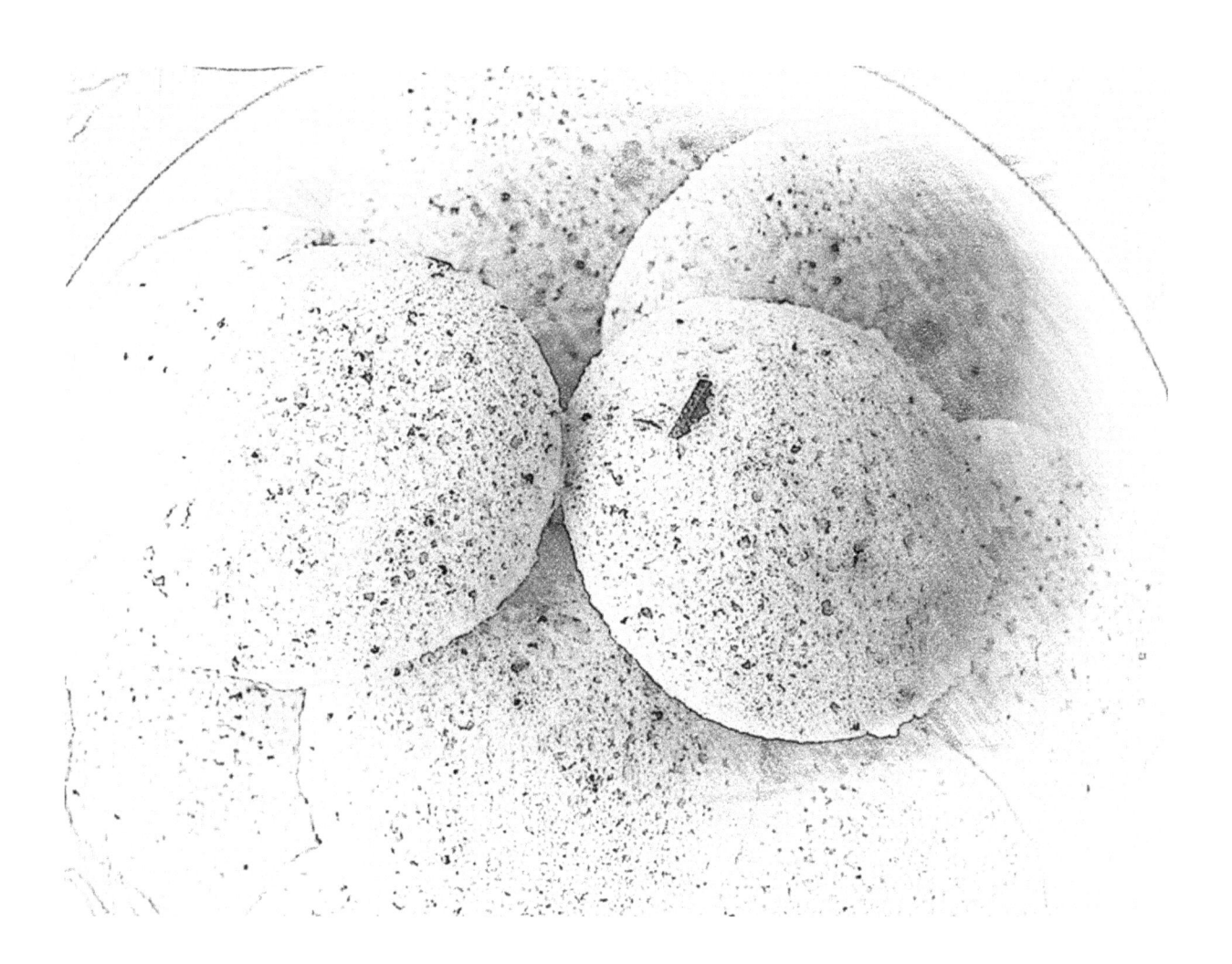

Ingredients:

For Rava Idli Batter:

- 1 cup fine semolina (rava or sooji)
- 1 cup plain yogurt (curd)
- 1/2 cup water (adjust as needed)
- 1/2 teaspoon mustard seeds
- 1/2 teaspoon cumin seeds
- 1/2 teaspoon chana dal (split chickpeas)
- 1/2 teaspoon urad dal (split black gram)
- A pinch of asafoetida (hing)
- 1-2 red chilies, finely cut (adjust to your spice preference)
- 1/2-inch piece of ginger, grated
- A few curry leaves, chopped
- 2 tablespoons oil
- 1/2 teaspoon baking soda (optional)
- Salt to taste

Instructions:

For Rava Idli Batter:

1. Heat 2 tablespoons of oil in a pan over medium heat. Add mustard seeds, cumin seeds, chana dal, urad dal, and a pinch of asafoetida. Sauté until the dals turn golden brown.
2. Add the chopped red chilies, grated ginger, and curry leaves. Sauté for another minute until the chilies become slightly soft.
3. Add the fine semolina (rava) to the pan. Roast it on low heat for about 5-7 minutes, or until the rava turns aromatic and changes color slightly. Be careful not to brown it too much; it should remain pale.

4. Remove the roasted rava from the heat and allow it to cool to room temperature.

5. Once the roasted rava has cooled, transfer it to a mixing bowl. Add yogurt and mix well to combine.

6. Gradually add water while stirring to achieve a thick but pourable batter. Ensure there are no lumps. Let the batter rest for about 15-20 minutes. The semolina will absorb the moisture and thicken during this time. If you prefer a slightly fluffier texture, you can add 1/2 teaspoon of baking soda to the batter at this stage. Mix well.

For Tempering:

- 1 tablespoon oil
- 1/2 teaspoon mustard seeds
- 1/2 teaspoon urad dal (split black gram)
- A few curry leaves

Instructions:

For Tempering:

1. Heat 1 tablespoon of oil in a small pan over medium heat. Add mustard seeds, urad dal, and curry leaves. Let the mustard seeds splutter and the dals turn golden brown.

2. Pour this tempering over the prepared Rava Idli batter. Mix well.

Steaming the Rava Idlis:

1. Grease the idli plates with a little oil or ghee.

2. Pour the Rava Idli batter into the greased idli molds.

3. Steam the idlis in a steamer or an idli maker for about 12-15 minutes, or until they are cooked through. You can check the doneness by inserting a toothpick or knife; it should come out clean.

4. Once done, remove the idlis from the molds using a spoon.

Serving Suggestions:

Potato saagu https://youtu.be/jlQ8FMdr7dA

Eggplant Saung https://youtu.be/9sCR3K0Eq3U

Ghee https://youtu.be/s6hL61F5BSQ

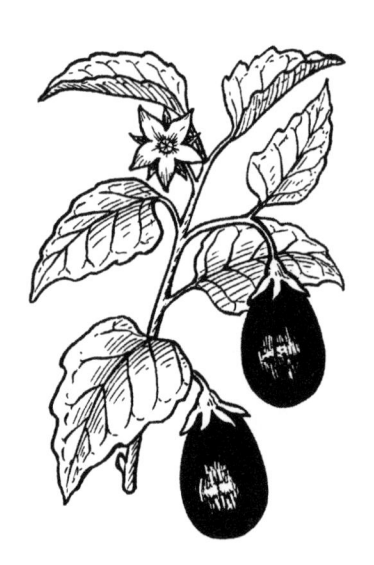

21. Sevai

Sevai is a popular South Indian dish made from steamed rice noodles. It can be served for breakfast, lunch, or dinner and is often accompanied by coconut chutney, sambar, or a variety of other side dishes.

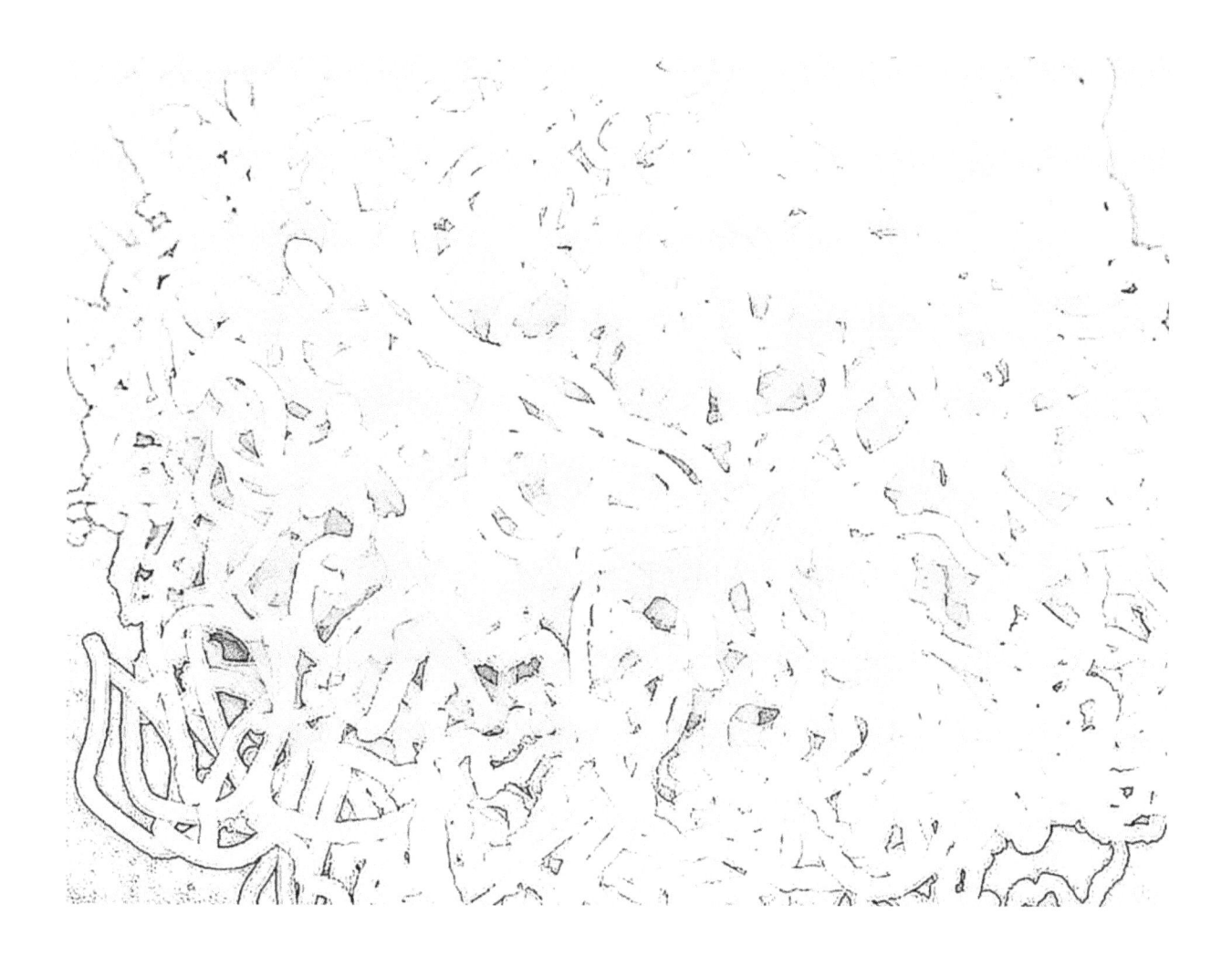

Ingredients:

For Making Sevai Dough:

- 1 cup rice flour
- 1 ¼ cups water
- ½ teaspoon oil
- ½ teaspoon salt

Instructions:

For making the Sevai dough:

1. In a saucepan, bring 1 1/4 cups of water to a boil. Add salt to the water.
2. Once the water is boiling, reduce the heat to low and add the rice flour. Stir quickly to combine and prevent lumps from forming.
3. Cook the mixture for 1-2 minutes on low heat, stirring continuously, until it forms a dough-like consistency. Turn off the heat.
4. Allow the dough to cool slightly until you can handle it comfortably. Knead the dough until it becomes smooth and soft.
5. Divide the dough into small portions and shape them into cylindrical logs. These logs will be used to make the rice noodles.
6. Grease the idli plates or a steamer tray with a little oil to prevent sticking. Place the cylindrical rice dough logs in the steamer and steam them for about 10-15 minutes until they become firm.
7. Once the steamed rice dough logs are cool enough to handle, grate them using a grater or a sevai press (also known as a "sevai nazhi" in Tamil) to form rice noodles.

This video shows how the hand pressed fresh noodles are made:

https://youtu.be/cocpHHGNq9M

Instructions for tempering Sevai:

- ½ teaspoon mustard seeds
- ½ teaspoon urad dal
- ½ teaspoon chana dal
- ½ teaspoon oil
- Asafoetida, a pinch
- 2 red chilis, broken
- Grated coconut
- Coriander leaves, chopped

---

1. Heat oil in a pan over medium heat. Add mustard seeds and let them splutter.
2. Add urad dal and chana dal. Sauté until the dals turn golden brown.
3. Add a pinch of asafoetida, chopped red chilies, and curry leaves. Sauté for a minute until the chilies become slightly soft.
4. Add the freshly grated rice noodles to the pan and mix gently.
5. Add salt to taste and continue to sauté for 2-3 minutes until everything is well combined and heated through.
6. Finally, add grated coconut and mix well.
7. Garnish with fresh coriander leaves if desired.

Serving Suggestions for Sevai:

Mor Kuzhambu https://youtu.be/V-1rGkmVsWM

Poricha Kuzhambu https://youtu.be/6D2AWP6STQo

Sampangi Pitlay https://youtu.be/n9qZ_EhkM-Q

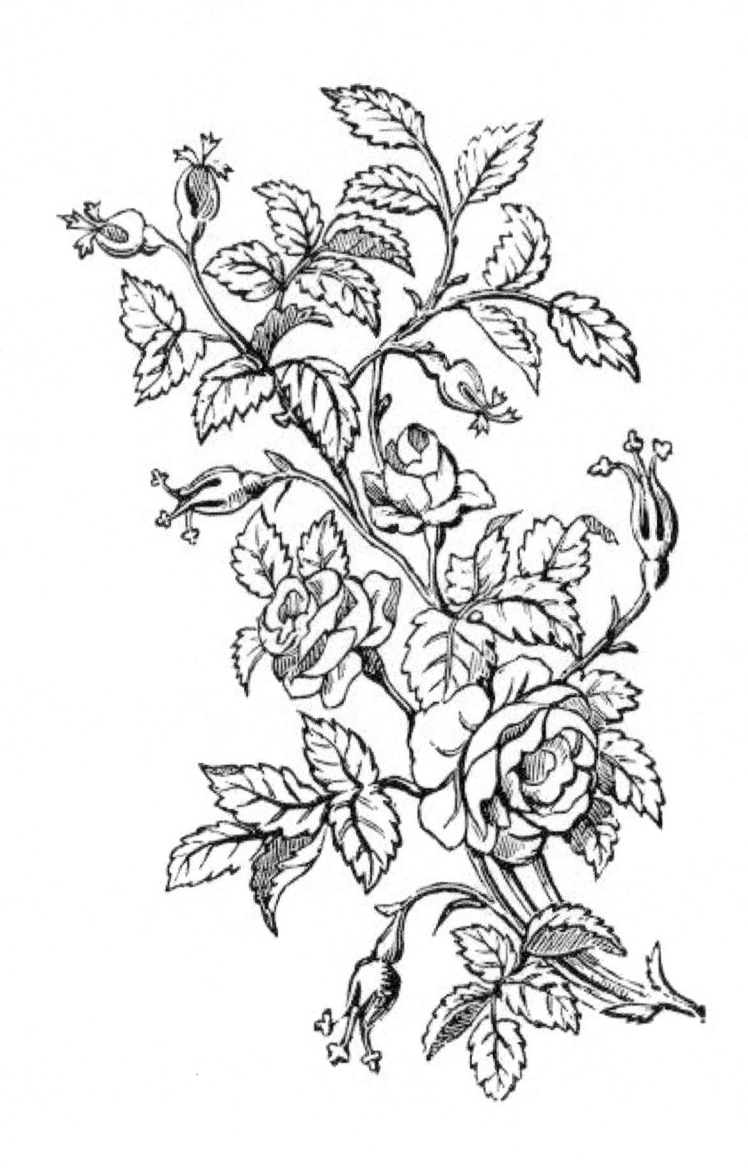

22. Thavalai Dosai

Thavalai Dosai, also known as Thavala Adai, is a traditional South Indian pancake made with a mixture of lentils and rice. It's known for its unique preparation method using a special utensil called a "thavalai" or "thavala," which is a shallow, wide, flat-bottomed vessel with depressions. Thavalai Dosai has a unique, rustic texture and a delicious mix of flavors from the lentils and spices. It's a wonderful South Indian dish that can be enjoyed for breakfast or as a snack.

Ingredients:

For making the Batter:

- 1 cup raw rice
- 1/2 cup parboiled rice (idli rice)
- 1/4 cup chana dal (split chickpeas)
- 1/4 cup toor dal (split pigeon peas)
- 1/4 cup urad dal (split black gram)
- 2-3 dried red chilies (adjust to your spice preference)
- 1/2 teaspoon asafoetida (hing)
- Salt to taste
- Water (for soaking and grinding)

Instructions:

To Prepare the Batter:

1. Wash the raw rice, parboiled rice, chana dal, toor dal, and urad dal together. Soak them in water for about 4-5 hours.
2. Drain the soaked ingredients and grind them into a coarse batter using minimal water. The batter should have a texture similar to that of regular dosa batter.
3. Add dried red chilies, asafoetida, and salt to the batter. Mix well.
4. Cover the batter and let it ferment for at least 4-6 hours or overnight. Fermentation is essential for the texture and flavor of Thavalai Dosai.

Ingredients:

For the Seasoning:

- 1 cup finely chopped green onions
- 2-3 red chilies, finely chopped
- A handful of chopped curry leaves
- 2 tablespoons finely chopped cilantro
- 1 tablespoon grated coconut (fresh or frozen)
- 1 teaspoon cumin seeds (jeera)
- Oil for cooking

Instructions:

For making Thavalai Dosai:

1. Heat a thavalai or any flat-bottomed shallow pan (like a cast-iron skillet) over medium heat. Grease it lightly with oil.
2. Once the pan is hot, reduce the heat to low. Pour a ladleful of batter into the center of the pan.
3. Using the back of the ladle, spread the batter in a circular motion to form a thick pancake. The pancake should have a slightly uneven surface.
4. Quickly sprinkle a portion of the chopped green onions, red chilies, curry leaves, cilantro, grated coconut, and cumin seeds over the pancake.
5. Drizzle a little oil around the edges and on top.
6. Cover the pan with a lid and cook on low heat until the bottom side turns golden brown and crispy. This should take about 5-7 minutes.

7. Carefully flip the Thavalai Dosai using a spatula and cook the other side until it's golden brown as well. Drizzle a little more oil if needed.

8. Remove the dosai from the pan and repeat the process with the remaining batter.

Serving Suggestions for Thavalai Dosai

Carrot chutney https://youtu.be/gtBSNX51YPg

Tomato gojju https://youtu.be/o3p_uB6btxaE

Saagu https://youtu.be/jlQ8FMdr7dA

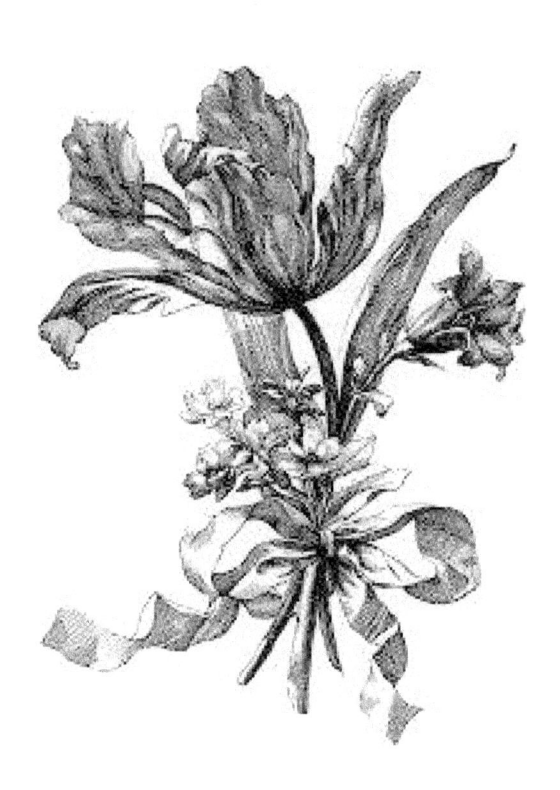

23. Thayir Vadai

Thayir Vadai, also known as Dahi Vada or Curd Vada, is a popular South Indian dish made from deep-fried lentil dumplings soaked in yogurt and topped with various seasonings and chutneys. It's a delicious and refreshing dish, especially on a hot day.

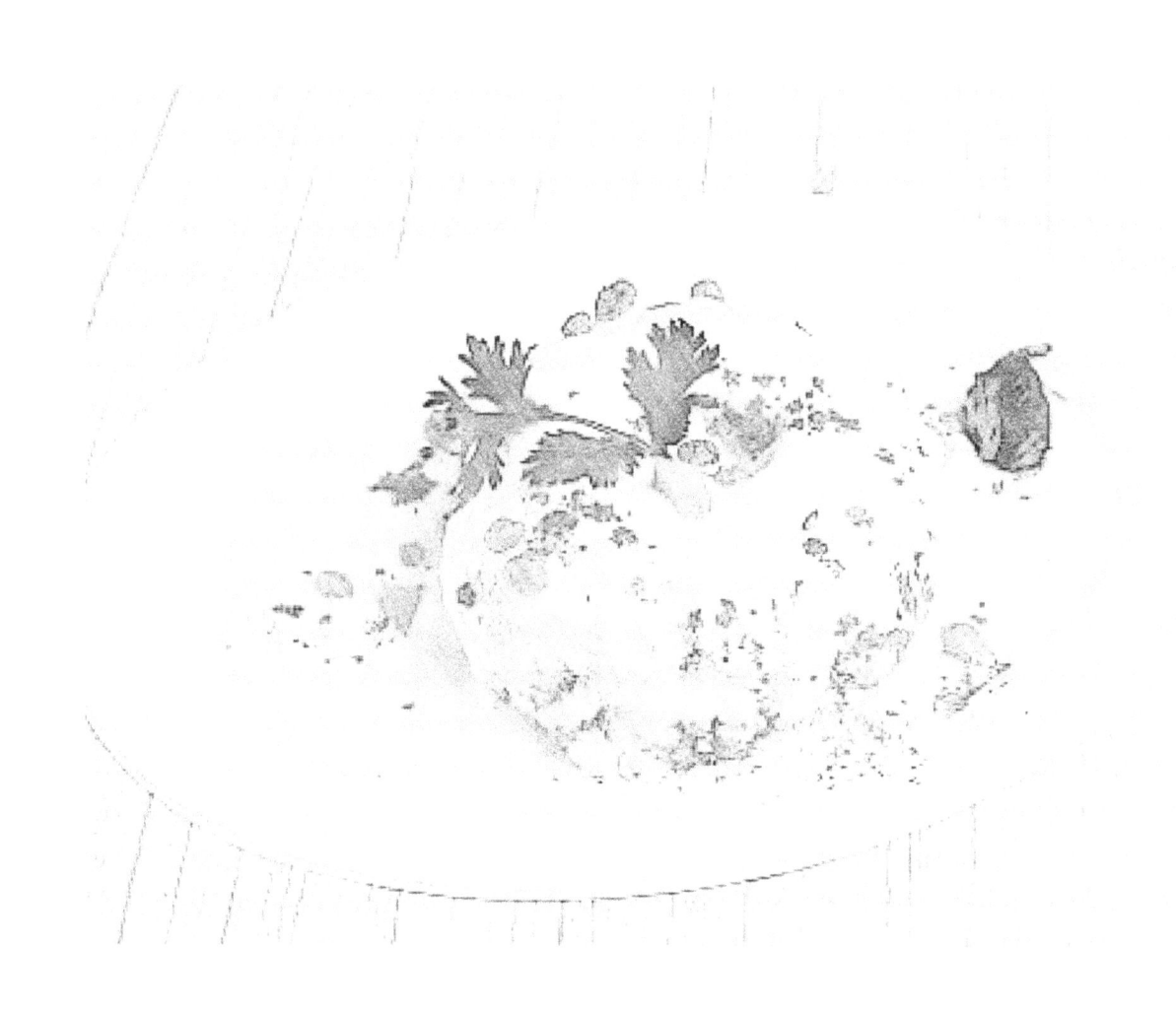

Ingredients:

For the Vada:

- 1 cup urad dal (split black gram)
- 2-3 red chilies, chopped (adjust to your spice preference)
- 1-inch piece of ginger, grated
- A pinch of asafoetida (hing)
- Salt to taste
- Oil for deep frying

Instructions:

To Make the Vada:

1. Wash the urad dal thoroughly under running water. Soak it in enough water for 3-4 hours.
2. Drain the soaked urad dal and grind it into a smooth batter using very little water. The batter should be thick and fluffy.
3. Add chopped red chilies, grated ginger, a pinch of asafoetida, and salt to the batter. Mix well.
4. Heat oil in a deep frying pan or kadai over medium heat.
5. Wet your hands and take a small portion of the batter. Flatten it slightly and make a hole in the center to form a vada shape.
6. Carefully slide the shaped vada into the hot oil. Fry the vadas in batches until they turn golden brown and crispy on both sides.
7. Remove the fried vadas from the oil and drain them on a paper towel to remove excess oil. Repeat this process for the remaining batter.

Ingredients:

For the Yogurt Mixture:

- 2 cups thick yogurt (curd)
- 1/2 cup water (adjust to achieve the desired consistency)
- Salt to taste
- ½ teaspoon toasted cumin seeds

Instructions:

For Preparing the Yogurt Mixture:

1. Whisk the thick yogurt until it becomes smooth and creamy. Add water gradually and continue whisking to achieve the desired consistency. The mixture should be slightly thinner than regular yogurt.
2. Season the yogurt mixture with salt and mix well.
3. Immerse the fried vadas in this yogurt mixture, ensuring they are fully coated. Allow them to soak for at least 20-30 minutes so that the vadas absorb the yogurt.

Ingredients:

For Seasoning:

- 1 tablespoon oil
- 1/2 teaspoon mustard seeds
- 1/2 teaspoon urad dal (split black gram)

- A few curry leaves
- 2-3 dried red chilies, broken into pieces
- A pinch of asafoetida (hing)

Instructions:

Seasoning the Thayir Vadai:

1. Heat 1 tablespoon of oil in a small pan over medium heat.
2. Add mustard seeds, urad dal, curry leaves, dried red chilies, and a pinch of asafoetida. Sauté until the mustard seeds start to splutter and the dals turn golden brown.
3. Pour this seasoning over the soaked vadas.

Ingredients:

For Garnish:

- Finely chopped coriander leaves
- Grated coconut (fresh or frozen)
- Red chili powder
- Tamarind chutney (optional)

Instructions:

For Garnish and Serve:

1. Garnish the Thayir Vadai with finely chopped coriander leaves, grated coconut, a sprinkle of red chili powder, and roasted cumin powder (if desired).
2. You can also drizzle some tamarind chutney for added flavor.
3. Serve chilled and enjoy your homemade Thayir Vadai!

Serving Suggestions:

Date Tamarind Chutney

https://thesattvicmethodcompany.com/sattvic-recipes/date-tamarind-chutney/

Cabbage - Ginger Chutney https://youtu.be/mxzOlZrUAlo

Tomato Gojju https://youtu.be/o3puB6btxaE

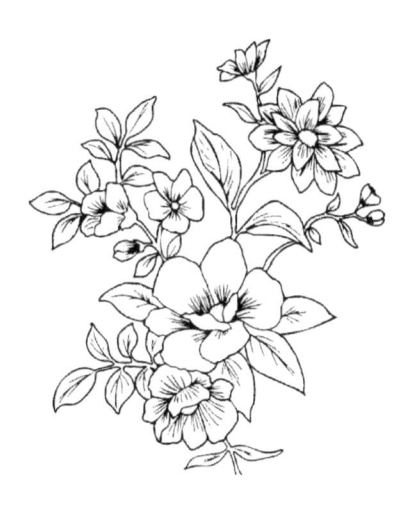

24. Tomato Upma

Tomato Upma is a popular South Indian dish made with semolina (known as rava or sooji) and tomatoes. It's a delicious and satisfying breakfast option.

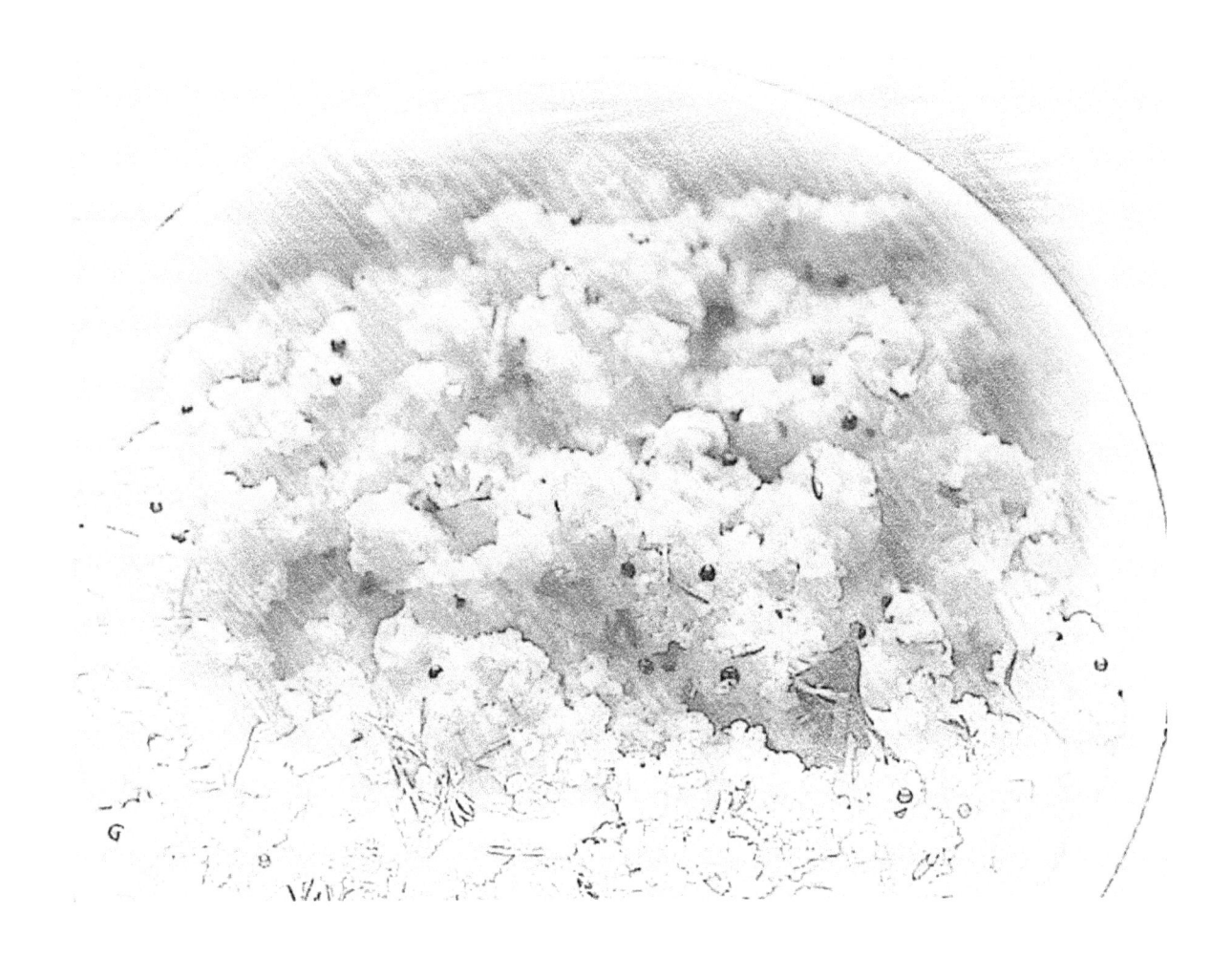

Ingredients:

- 1 cup semolina (rava or sooji)
- 2 tablespoons ghee (clarified butter) or coconut oil for a vegan option
- 1 teaspoon cumin seeds
- 1/2 teaspoon black mustard seeds
- 1/2 teaspoon urad dal (split black gram)
- 1/2 teaspoon chana dal (split chickpeas)
- 1/4 cup chopped cashew nuts (optional)
- 1 medium-sized green onion bunch, finely chopped
- 2-3 red chilies, finely chopped (adjust to your spice preference)
- 1-inch piece of ginger, grated
- 2 ripe tomatoes, finely chopped
- A pinch of asafoetida (hing)
- A few curry leaves
- 2 cups of water
- Salt to taste
- Fresh coriander leaves for garnish

Instructions:

1. Heat a dry skillet or pan over medium heat. Add the semolina and roast it for about 4-5 minutes or until it turns fragrant and slightly golden. Be careful not to over-roast; it should not turn brown. Remove it from the pan and set it aside.
2. In the same pan, heat the ghee or coconut oil over medium heat.
3. Add the cumin seeds, black mustard seeds, urad dal, and chana dal. Sauté until the dals turn golden brown and the mustard seeds start to pop.

4. If using cashew nuts, add them and sauté until they turn golden. Then, add the finely chopped onion, red chilies, grated ginger, and curry leaves. Sauté until the onions become translucent.
5. Add the finely chopped tomatoes and cook for about 3-4 minutes until they soften.
6. Add a pinch of asafoetida and the roasted semolina to the pan. Mix everything together.
7. Carefully pour in 2 cups of water while continuously stirring to avoid lumps. Stir well to combine.
8. Reduce the heat to low, cover the pan with a lid, and let the Upma simmer for about 3-4 minutes, or until the semolina has absorbed all the water and is cooked through.
9. Season the Tomato Upma with salt to taste and mix well.
10. Garnish the Tomato Upma with fresh coriander leaves. Remove it from the heat.
11. Tomato Upma is best served hot. It can be enjoyed on its own or with coconut chutney.

Serving Suggestions:

Tomato Upma is best served with

Raita https://youtu.be/Svd7w-MsLd8

Apple thokku https://youtu.be/kLpvFTfA4Qk

Ghee https://youtu.be/s6hL61F5BSQ

25. Uthappam

Uthappam is a popular South Indian dish that is essentially a thick, savory pancake made from fermented rice and urad dal (black gram) batter. It's often topped with various ingredients like chopped vegetables and is cooked on a griddle until it's crispy on the outside and soft on the inside.

Ingredients:

For Uthappam Batter:

- 1 cup idli rice or regular rice
- 1/4 cup urad dal (black gram)
- 1/4 teaspoon fenugreek seeds (optional)
- Salt to taste
- Water for grinding

Instructions:

To make Uthappam Batter:

1. Wash the rice, urad dal, and fenugreek seeds together thoroughly and soak them in water separately for about 4-6 hours.
2. Drain the soaked rice and urad dal. Then, grind them separately into a smooth paste using as little water as possible. The batter should be thick.
3. Mix the rice and urad dal batters together in a large bowl. Add salt and mix well.
4. Allow the batter to ferment overnight or for at least 6-8 hours. The fermentation time may vary depending on the temperature of your surroundings. The batter should rise and become slightly frothy when it's ready.

Ingredients:

For Topping (Optional):

- Finely chopped vegetables like tomatoes, bell peppers, and cilantro
- Grated coconut (fresh or frozen)
- Sesame seeds
- Curry leaves

For Cooking:

- Oil or ghee for cooking

Making Uthappam:

1. Heat a non-stick griddle or dosa pan over medium heat. Grease it lightly with oil or ghee.
2. Pour a ladleful of the fermented batter onto the center of the griddle. Using the back of the ladle, spread the batter in a circular motion to make a thick pancake. Uthappam is thicker than dosa, so don't spread it too thin.
3. Quickly sprinkle your desired toppings on top of the Uthappam - chopped vegetables, grated coconut, sesame seeds, and curry leaves work well.
4. Drizzle a little oil or ghee around the edges of the Uthappam and a few drops on top.
5. Cover the griddle with a lid and cook on medium-low heat until the Uthappam's bottom side turns golden brown and crisp. It should take about 3-4 minutes.

6. Flip the Uthappam and cook the other side until it's golden brown and cooked through, about 2-3 minutes.

7. Remove the Uthappam from the griddle and serve hot.

Serving Suggestions:

Parsley chutney https://youtu.be/ADth8ETWRR8

Molagapodi https://youtu.be/yyN9cssAoZo

Potatoes in Tamarind Gravy https://youtu.be/iUA3ezXjjU0

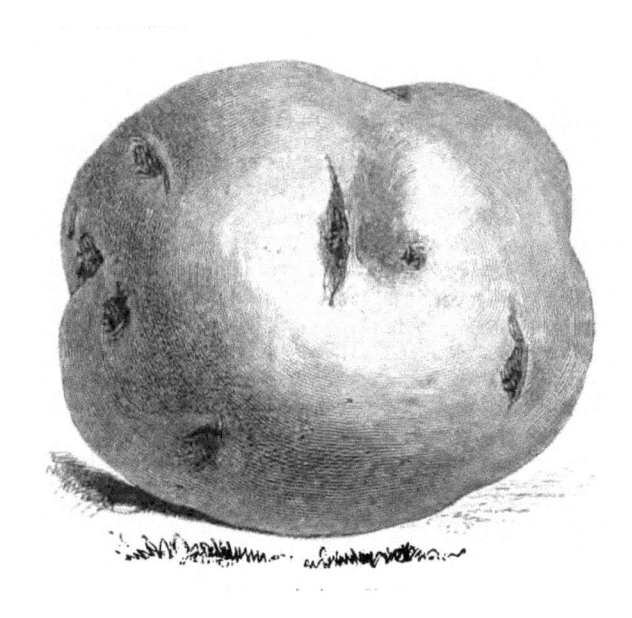

26. Ven Pongal

Ven Pongal is a traditional South Indian dish made with rice and lentils, flavored with black pepper, cumin, and ghee. It's often served as a savory breakfast dish, and it's simple to make. Ven Pongal is traditionally served with coconut chutney and sambar. It's a comforting and filling breakfast dish with a wonderful combination of flavors from the spices and ghee.

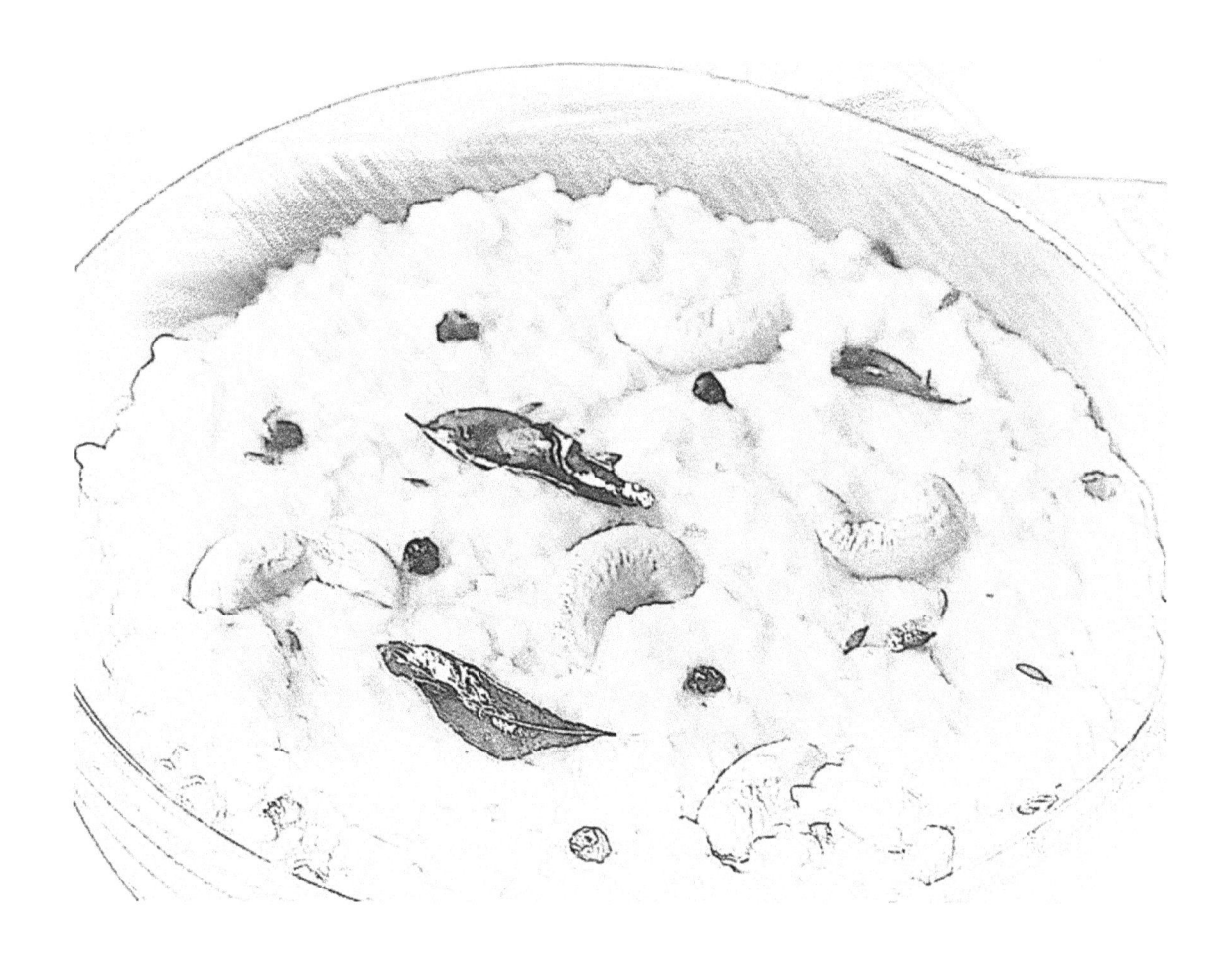

Ingredients:

- 1 cup raw rice
- ¼ cup split yellow moong dal (lentils)
- 2 tablespoons ghee (clarified butter)
- 1 teaspoon cumin seeds
- 1 teaspoon black pepper, coarsely crushed
- ½ teaspoon grated ginger
- A pinch of asafoetida (hing)
- A few curry leaves
- 2-3 red chilies, slit lengthwise (adjust to your spice preference)
- 2-3 tablespoons cashew nuts (optional)
- Salt to taste
- Water
- Fresh curry leaves for garnish

Instructions:

1. Wash the rice and moong dal together under running water until the water runs clear. Soak them in enough water for about 30 minutes. Then, drain the water.

2. *Cook Rice and Lentils:*
    - In a pressure cooker, add the soaked and drained rice and moong dal.
    - Add 4 cups of water and a pinch of asafoetida.
    - Close the lid without the weight and cook on medium heat for 2-3 whistles or until the rice and lentils are soft and well-cooked. If you don't have a pressure cooker, you can cook them in a regular pot, but it will take longer.

3. In a separate pan, heat the ghee over medium heat.
    - Add the cumin seeds and let them splutter.

- Add the coarsely crushed black pepper, grated ginger, curry leaves, and red chilies. Sauté for a minute or until the chilies become slightly soft.
- If using cashew nuts, add them and sauté until they turn golden.

4. *Combine the Tempering:*
    - Once the rice and lentils in the pressure cooker have cooked and the pressure has released, open the lid.
    - Pour the tempered mixture (ghee and spices) into the cooked rice and lentils. Mix well.
5. Add salt to taste and mix again. Adjust the salt to your preference.
6. Garnish with fresh curry leaves. Your Ven Pongal is ready to be served hot.

Serving Suggestions:

Tomato gojju https://youtu.be/o3puB6btxaE

Apple thokku https://youtu.be/kwH-X7zUiXg

Zucchini-cumin https://youtu.be/4Ob8Oq-f6i8

27. Vangibaath

Vangibaath is a flavorful South Indian rice dish made with brinjals (eggplants) and a special spice blend known as "vangibaath masala." This freshly spiced Vangibaath is a delightful dish with a rich blend of flavors and the goodness of eggplants. Making it with fresh spices enhances the taste and aroma.

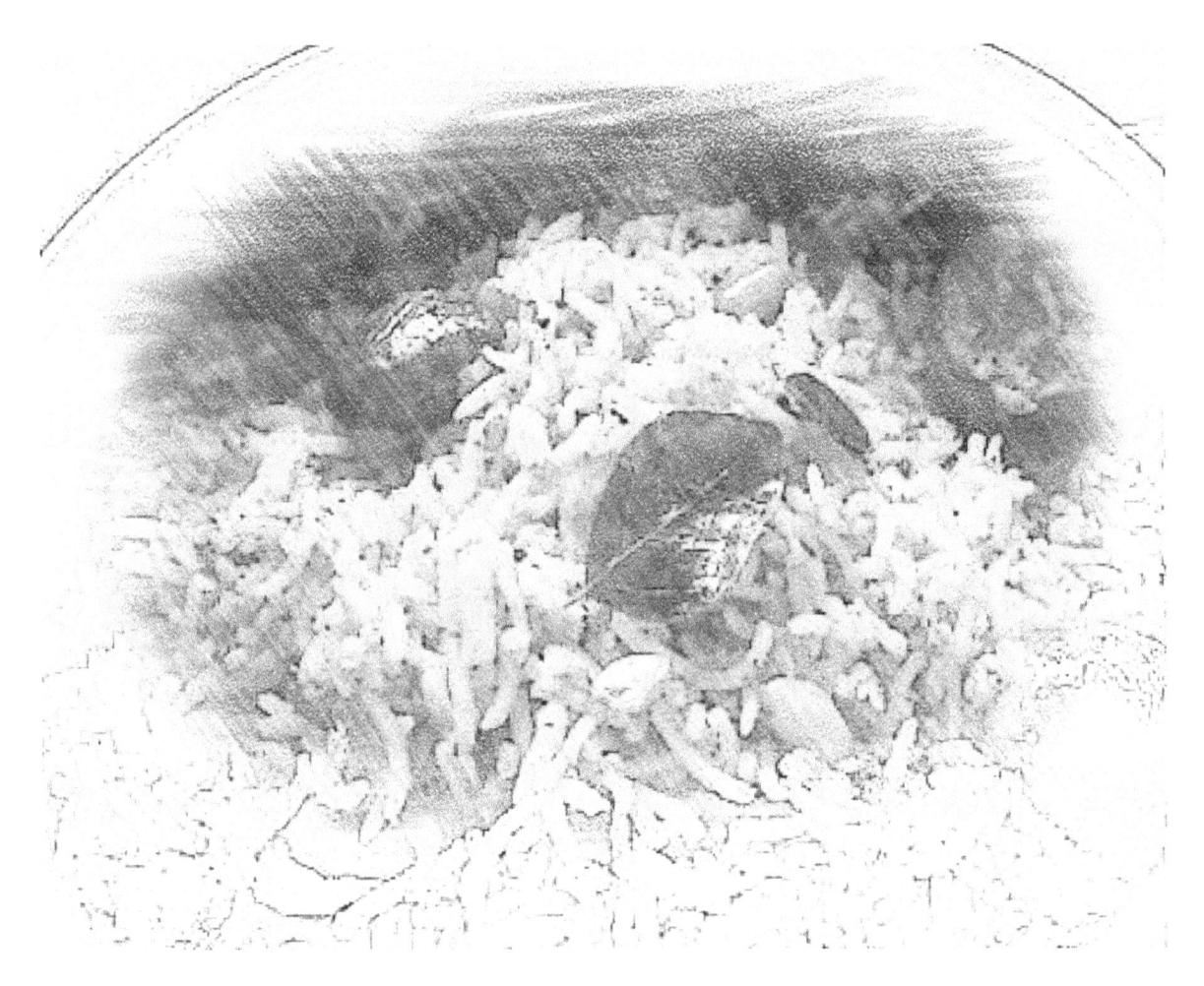

Ingredients:

For Vangibaath Masala:

- 1 teaspoon coriander seeds
- 1/2 teaspoon cumin seeds
- 1/2 teaspoon fenugreek seeds
- 1/2 teaspoon mustard seeds
- 4-5 dried red chilies (adjust to your spice preference)
- 1 tablespoon grated coconut (fresh or frozen)
- A small piece of tamarind (about 1/2 teaspoon tamarind paste)
- 1 tablespoons oil for roasting the spices

Instructions:

To make Vangibaath Masala:

1. Heat a pan on medium-low heat. Add the coriander seeds, cumin seeds, fenugreek seeds, mustard seeds, dried red chilies, grated coconut, and tamarind.
2. Dry roast the spices until they become fragrant and the coconut turns light golden. Stir frequently to prevent burning. This should take about 5-7 minutes.
3. Allow the roasted ingredients to cool, then grind them into a fine paste using a little water. Set aside.

Ingredients:

To make Vangibaath:

- 1 cup long-grain rice (like Basmati), washed and drained
- 1 1/2 cups diced brinjals (eggplants), about 2 small eggplants
- 1 teaspoon mustard seeds
- 1/2 teaspoon urad dal (split black gram)
- 1/2 teaspoon chana dal (split chickpeas)
- 1/4 cup raw peanuts
- A pinch of asafoetida (hing)
- A few curry leaves
- 1/4 teaspoon turmeric powder
- Salt to taste
- Fresh coriander leaves for garnish
- 2 tablespoons oil

Instructions:

Make Vangibaath:

1. Heat 2 tablespoons of oil in a large, heavy-bottomed pan or kadai over medium heat.
2. Add mustard seeds, urad dal, and chana dal. Sauté until the dals turn golden brown and the mustard seeds start to pop.
3. Add peanuts and sauté for another 2-3 minutes until they begin to turn golden.
4. Add a pinch of asafoetida, curry leaves, and diced brinjals. Cook for about 7-8 minutes until the brinjals become tender and slightly caramelized.
5. Add turmeric powder and salt. Mix well.

6. Add the ground Vangi Bath masala paste and sauté for a couple of minutes until the oil starts to separate from the masala.
7. Add the washed and drained rice. Mix everything together gently, ensuring that the rice is coated with the masala.
8. Add 2 cups of water and bring it to a boil. Reduce the heat to low, cover, and simmer for about 15-20 minutes or until the rice is cooked and the water is absorbed. If the rice is not fully cooked, add a little more water and continue to simmer.
9. Once the rice is done, remove from heat and let it sit for 5 minutes before fluffing it with a fork.
10. Garnish with fresh coriander leaves and serve hot.

Serving Suggestions:

Raita https://youtu.be/Svd7w-MsLd8

Salad https://youtu.be/enjODTQPsBU

Cabbage pakoda https://youtu.be/vY4jSb13fGI

28. Wheat Rava Pongal

Wheat Rava Pongal is a nutritious and delicious South Indian dish that's often served for breakfast or as a light meal. It's made using wheat semolina (wheat rava) instead of the traditional rice, making it a healthier alternative.

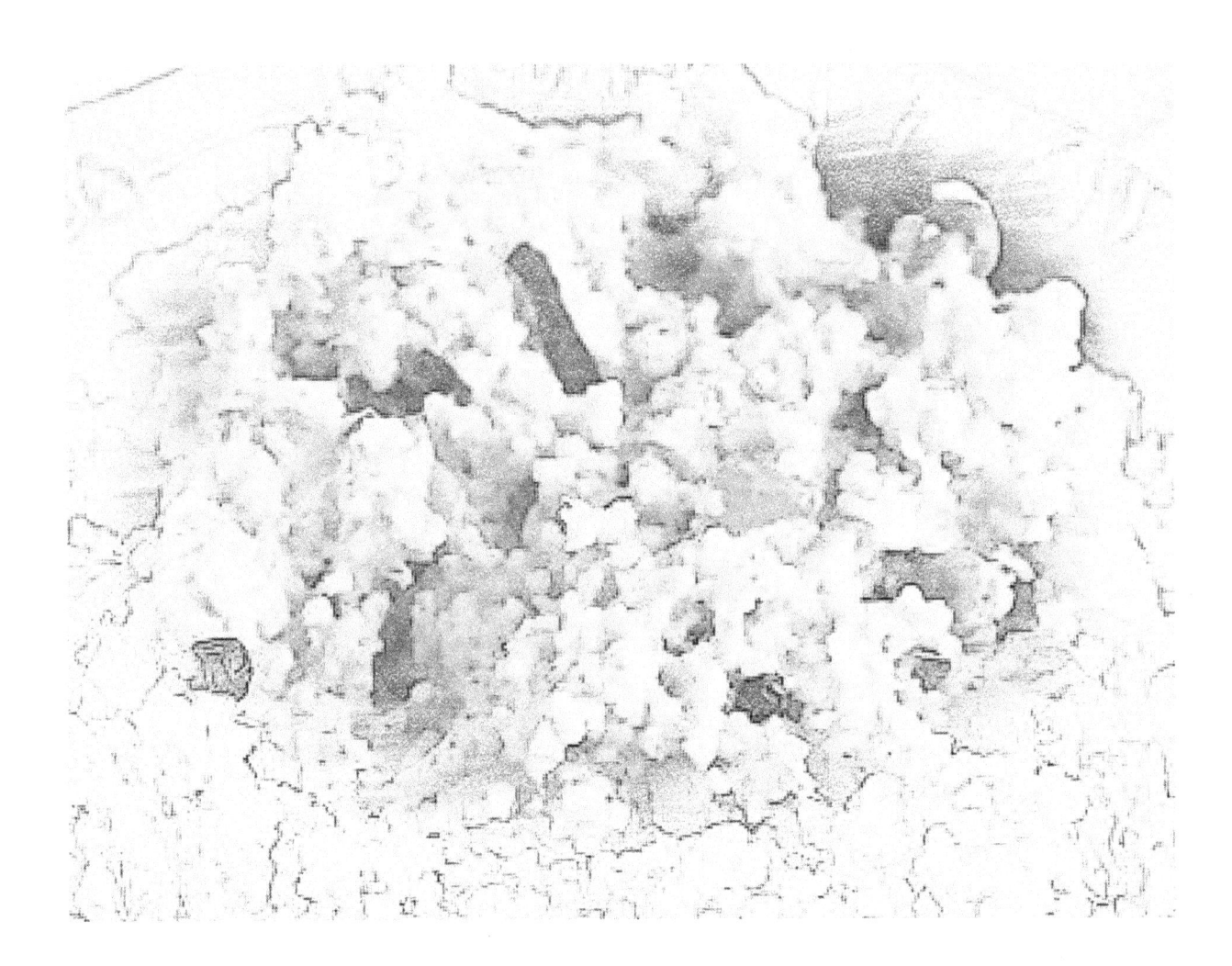

Ingredients:

To make Pongal:

- 1 cup wheat rava (wheat semolina)
- 1/4 cup yellow split moong dal (lentils)
- 2 1/2 cups water
- 1/2 teaspoon black pepper corns
- 1/2 teaspoon cumin seeds
- 1/2 inch piece of ginger, finely grated
- 1-2 red chilies, finely chopped (adjust to your spice preference)
- A pinch of asafoetida (hing)
- A few curry leaves
- 2 tablespoons ghee or clarified butter
- Salt to taste

For Tempering:

- 1 tablespoon ghee or clarified butter
- 1 teaspoon mustard seeds
- 1 teaspoon cumin seeds
- 1-2 dried red chilies (break them into pieces)
- A pinch of asafoetida (hing)

Instructions:

1. Wash the yellow split moong dal under running water until the water runs clear. Drain and set aside.

2. In a dry skillet or pan, roast the wheat rava over medium heat until it turns slightly golden and emits a nutty aroma. This takes about 3-4 minutes. Transfer it to a plate and set aside.

3. In a pressure cooker or a pot, add the roasted wheat rava, washed lentils, water, black pepper, cumin seeds, grated ginger, chopped red chilies, asafoetida, and a few curry leaves. Close the lid of the pressure cooker (without the weight) or the pot and cook for 2-3 whistles or until the lentils are soft and well-cooked.

4. In a separate small pan, heat 1 tablespoon of ghee. Add the mustard seeds and let them splutter. Add the cumin seeds, dried red chilies, and a pinch of asafoetida. Fry for a few seconds until the spices are fragrant.

5. Once the pressure cooker has depressurized and you can open it safely, open the lid and add the tempered spices to the cooked pongal. Mix well.

6. Add 2 tablespoons of ghee to the pongal and salt to taste. Mix everything thoroughly. Adjust the salt and ghee according to your taste preferences.

7. Your Wheat Rava Pongal is ready to be served. Enjoy!

Serving Suggestions:

Raita https://youtu.be/Svd7w-MsLd8

Gojju https://youtu.be/o3puB6btxaE

Chickpea stew https://youtu.be/dnxs3xQpf6U

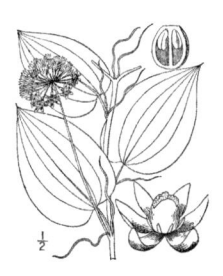

29. Yellu chadam

Yellu Chadam, also known as Sesame Rice, is a traditional South Indian dish known for its nutty and aromatic flavor. It's a delicious and easy-to-make recipe that's perfect for lunch or dinner. Yellu Chadam makes for a delightful and flavorful meal. You can enjoy it on its own or with a side of yogurt or pickle. It's a wonderful way to incorporate the rich taste of sesame into your meal.

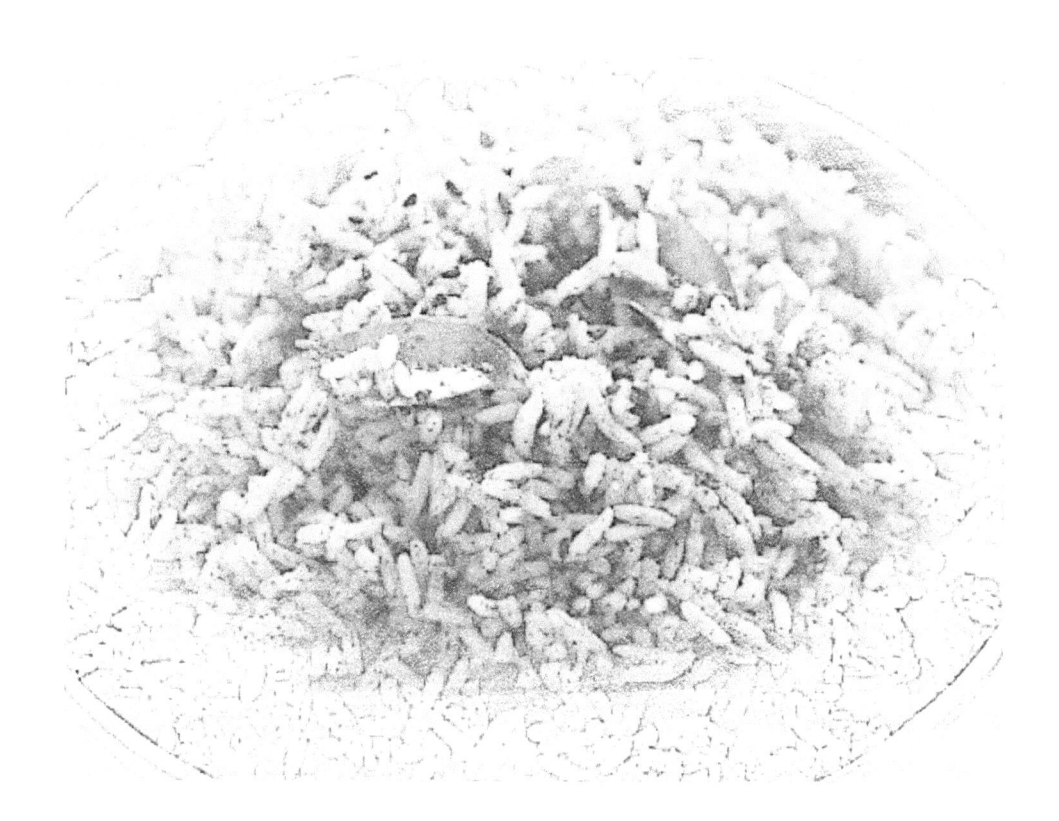

Ingredients:

For Sesame Paste:

- 1/2 cup white sesame seeds
- 2-3 dried red chilies (adjust to your spice preference)
- 2 tablespoons grated coconut (optional)
- A small piece of tamarind (about 1/2 teaspoon tamarind pulp)
- Salt to taste

Instructions:

Preparing Sesame Paste:

1. Heat a dry skillet or pan over medium heat. Add the white sesame seeds and roast them, stirring continuously, until they turn light golden brown and release a nutty aroma. Be cautious not to burn them.
2. Let the roasted sesame seeds cool for a few minutes. Then, transfer them to a blender or spice grinder. Add dried red chilies, grated coconut (if using), tamarind, and salt. Grind

this mixture into a smooth paste using as little water as possible. The paste should be thick and creamy. Set it aside.

For Yellu Chadam:

- 1 cup rice (preferably short-grain rice like sona masuri)
- 2 tablespoons sesame oil (you can use regular cooking oil as well)
- ½ teaspoon mustard seeds
- ½ teaspoon urad dal (black gram lentils
- ½ teaspoon chana dal
- A pinch of asafoetida (hing)
- A few curry leaves
- 1-2 dried red chilies, broken into pieces
- Salt to taste

Instructions:

Cooking Yellu Chadam:

1. Cook the rice as you normally would, either by boiling or using a rice cooker. Make sure the rice grains are separate and not too sticky. Allow it to cool slightly.
2. In a large, deep skillet or pan, heat sesame oil over medium heat. Add mustard seeds and allow them to splutter. Then, add urad dal, chana dal, dried red chilies, asafoetida, and curry leaves. Sauté until the dals turn golden brown.

3. Lower the heat and add the prepared sesame paste to the skillet. Stir well to combine with the tempering. Cook this mixture for a couple of minutes, allowing the sesame flavors to meld with the tempering.
4. Add the cooked and slightly cooled rice to the skillet. Gently mix the rice with the sesame paste and tempering. Ensure that the rice is evenly coated with the sesame paste.
5. Taste the Yellu Chadam and adjust salt and spiciness according to your preference. If you want it spicier, you can add more dried red chilies at this stage.
6. Yellu Chadam is ready to be served. It's traditionally served at room temperature or slightly warm.

Serving Suggestions:

Yogurt

Ghee https://youtu.be/s6hL61F5BSQ

Cabbage-ginger chutney https://youtu.be/mxzOlZrUAlo

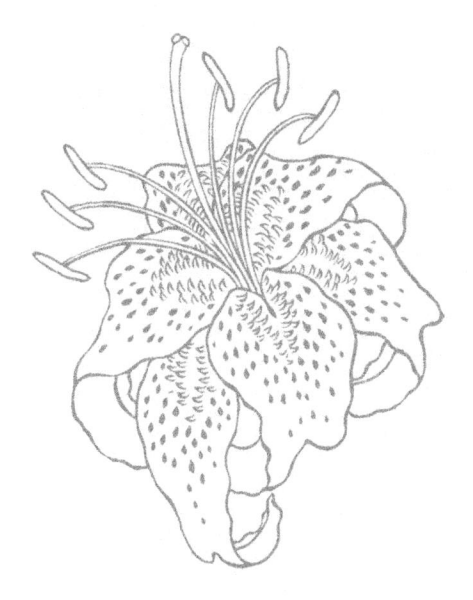

30. Yelimichai Chadam

Also known as Lemon Rice, is a popular South Indian dish known for its tangy and refreshing flavor. It's a quick and easy recipe that's perfect for a light lunch or as a side dish for festivals and gatherings. Yelimichai Chadam is a versatile dish that's perfect for picnics, tiffin boxes, and potlucks. Its zesty and tangy flavor makes it a favorite among people of all ages. Enjoy this delightful South Indian classic!

Ingredients:

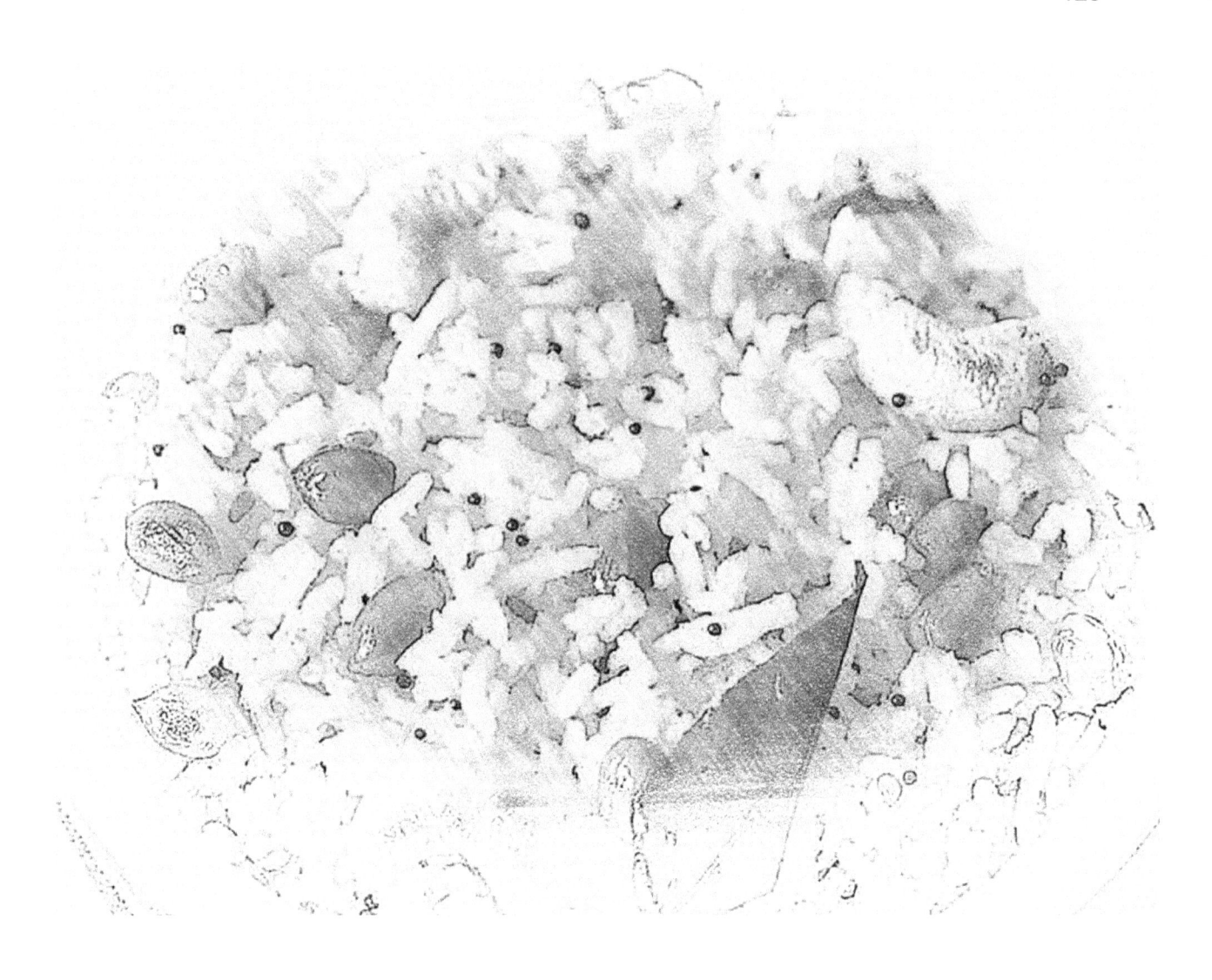

- 1 cup cooked rice (preferably short-grain rice like sona masuri)
- 2 tablespoons vegetable oil
- 1/2 teaspoon mustard seeds
- 1/2 teaspoon urad dal (black gram lentils)
- 1/2 teaspoon chana dal (split chickpeas)
- A pinch of asafoetida (hing)

- 2-3 dried red chilies, broken into pieces (adjust to your spice preference)
- 10-12 curry leaves
- 1/4 cup roasted peanuts
- 2-3 tablespoons lemon juice (adjust to taste)
- 1/2 teaspoon turmeric powder
- Salt to taste
- Fresh coriander leaves, chopped, for garnish (optional)

Instructions:

1. Cook the rice according to your preferred method. Make sure the rice is cooked well and the grains are separate. Allow it to cool slightly.
2. **Tempering:** In a large, deep skillet or pan, heat vegetable oil over medium heat. Add mustard seeds and allow them to splutter. Then, add urad dal, chana dal, dried red chilies, asafoetida, and curry leaves. Sauté until the dals turn golden brown.
3. **Adding Peanuts:** Add the roasted peanuts to the skillet and sauté for a couple of minutes until they become crisp.
4. Add turmeric powder and salt to the skillet. Mix well to evenly distribute the spices.
5. Lower the heat and add the cooked rice to the skillet. Gently mix the rice with the tempering and spices, ensuring that the rice is well coated.
6. Drizzle the lemon juice over the rice and give it a good stir. Adjust the amount of lemon juice according to your taste preference. The lemon juice should provide a tangy and refreshing flavor.

7. Taste the Yelimichai Chadam and adjust the salt and lemon juice if needed. You can also add more red chilies for extra spiciness.

8. If desired, garnish the lemon rice with fresh chopped coriander leaves for added freshness and flavor.

9. Yelimichai Chadam is ready to be served.

Serving Suggestions-

Sattvic Apple Thokku https://youtu.be/kLpvFTfA4Qk

Parsley Chutney https://youtu.be/ADth8ETWRR8

Okra Crisps https://youtu.be/CmdiI1T3stk

List of ingredients used in the book

- Asafoetida
- Baking soda
- Banana
- Black peppercorn
- Cardamom powder
- Cashew nuts
- Chickpeas
- Chilies, dry
- Coconut
- Coriander, cilantro
- Curry leaf
- Doenjang
- Eggplant
- Ghee
- Ginger
- Green Peas
- Jeera, cumin seeds
- Lime juice
- Maida, All purpose flour
- Mango
- Miso sauce
- Mixed Vegetables
- Moong dal, mung beans
- Mustard seeds
- Oil
- Papaya
- Peanuts, roasted
- Poha, flat rice
- Potato
- Raisins
- Rice, flour
- Rice, parboiled
- Rice, raw
- Saffron
- Salt
- Semolina, cream of wheat
- Sugar
- Tamarind pulp
- Tomato
- Toor dal, pigeon pea
- Turmeric powder
- Urad dal, black gram
- Water
- Yeast
- Yogurt

Stocking your Sattvic Pantry

Essentials

- Non-fluoridated water
- Wild or brown Rice (grain and flour)
- All-purpose flour or maida
- Farina or Rava or Suji
- Oats
- Wheat (flour)
- Millet (grain and flour)
- Flat rice
- Raw cane sugar
- Jaggery
- Mung beans
- Toor dal

- Garbanzo beansPink salt
- Mango powder or Amchur
- Turmeric powder
- Coriander seeds
- Fenugreek seeds
- Cumin seeds
- Sesame seeds
- Peanut
- Flax seeds
- Sunflower seeds
- Coconut oil
- Red Chilies

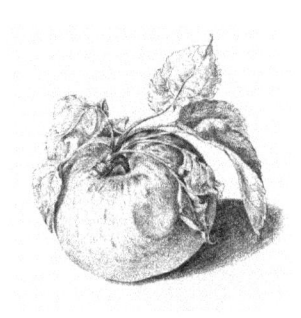

Your Sattvic Pantry

Fresh stock

Organic, grassfed, non violent source of milk, yogurt, and butter

- Yogurt
- Vegetables
- Fruits
- Coconut

- Cilantro
- Curry leaves
- Lime or lemon
- Ginger

Condiments

- Cardamom
- Cashew nuts
- Raisins

- Saffron
- Cloves
- Ginger powder

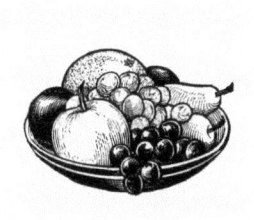

Other Sattvic Cookbooks

https://thesattvicmethodcompany.com/product-category/books/

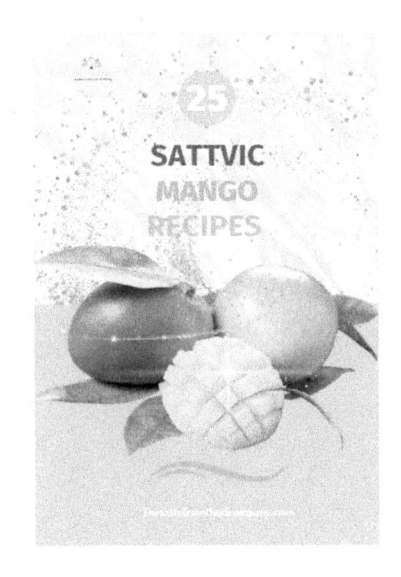

Mango Recipes

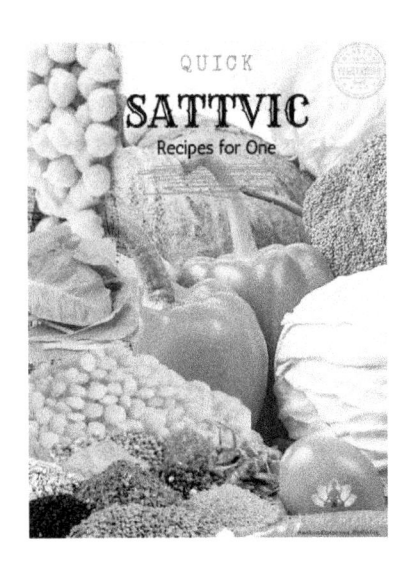

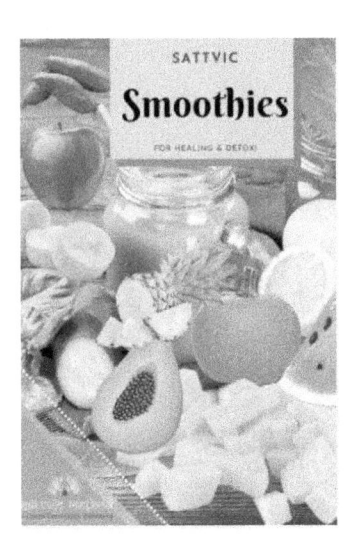

Smoothies

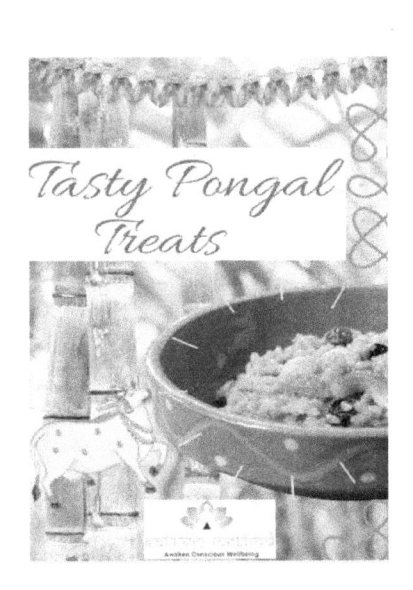

Quick Sattvic Recipes for one

Pongal Treats

135

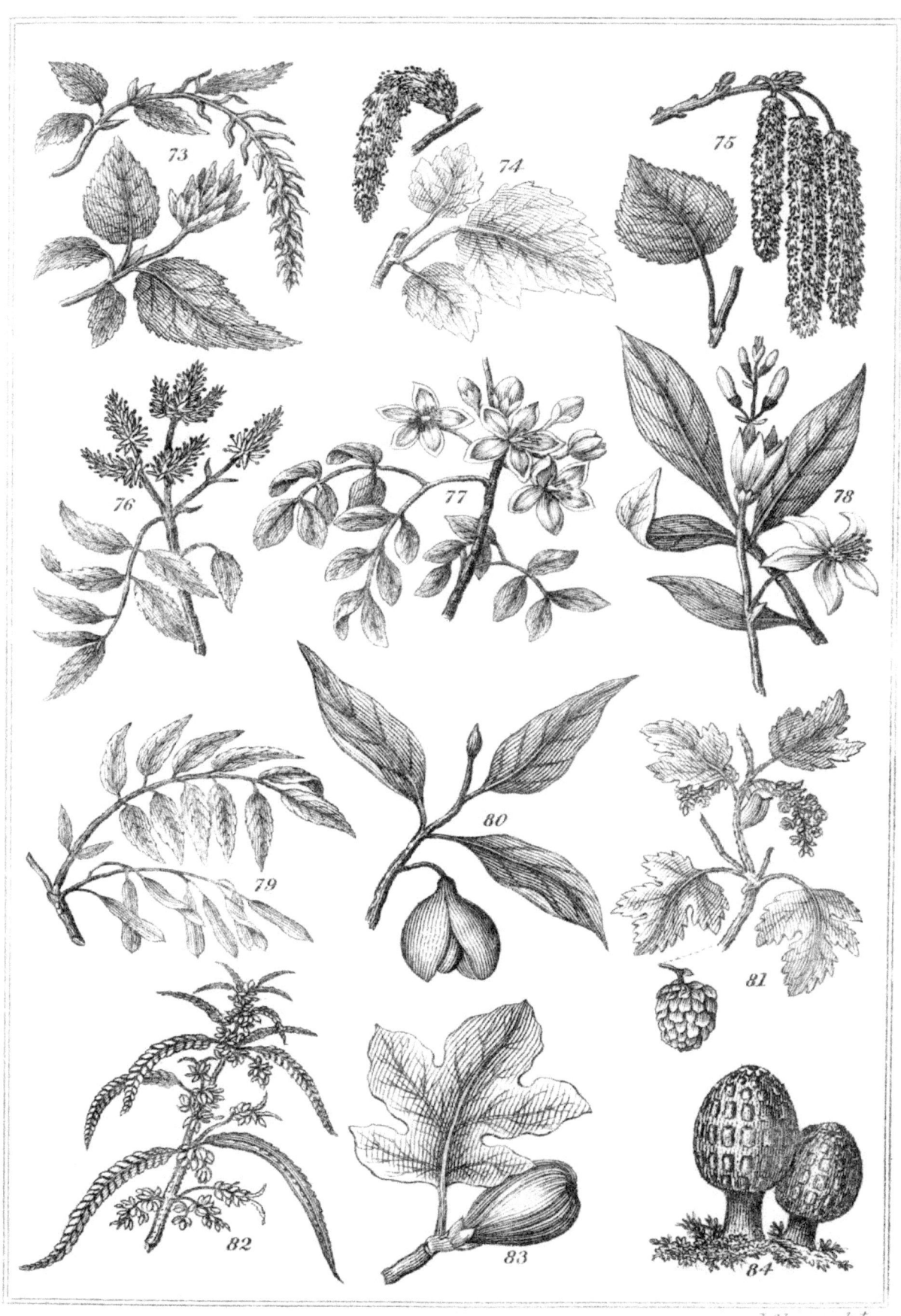

VEGETABLES.

Milton Keynes UK
Ingram Content Group UK Ltd.
UKHW050710220124
436466UK00017B/747